Geriatric Psychiatry

Editors

DAN G. BLAZER
SUSAN K. SCHULTZ

PSYCHIATRIC CLINICS
OF NORTH AMERICA

www.psych.theclinics.com

March 2018 • Volume 41 • Number 1

ELSEVIER

1600 John F. Kennedy Boulevard • Suite 1800 • Philadelphia, Pennsylvania, 19103-2899

http://www.theclinics.com

PSYCHIATRIC CLINICS OF NORTH AMERICA Volume 41, Number 1
March 2018 ISSN 0193-953X, ISBN-13: 978-0-323-58170-7

Editor: Lauren Boyle
Developmental Editor: Kristen Helm

Psychiatric Clinics of North America (ISSN 0193-953X) is published quarterly by Elsevier Inc., 360 Park Avenue South, New York, NY 10010-1710. Months of issue are March, June, September, and December. Business and Editorial Offices: 1600 John F. Kennedy Blvd., Suite 1800, Philadelphia, PA 19103-2899. Periodicals postage paid at New York, NY and additional mailing offices. Subscription prices are $321.00 per year (US individuals), $666.00 per year (US institutions), $100.00 per year (US students/residents), $391.00 per year (Canadian individuals), $460.00 per year (international individuals), $838.00 per year (Canadian & international institutions), and $220.00 per year (Canadian & international students/residents). Foreign air speed delivery is included in all *Clinics'* subscription prices. All prices are subject to change without notice. **POSTMASTER:** Send address changes to *Psychiatric Clinics of North America*, Elsevier Health Sciences Division, Subscription Customer Service, 3251 Riverport Lane, Maryland Heights, MO 63043. **Customer Service: 1-800-654-2452 (US). From outside the United States, call 1-314-447-8871. Fax: 1-314-447-8029. E-mail: journalscustomerservice-usa@elsevier.com (for print support) and journalsonline support-usa@elsevier.com (for online support).**

Reprints. For copies of 100 or more, of articles in this publication, please contact the Commercial Reprints Department, Elsevier Inc., 360 Park Avenue South, New York, New York 10010-1710. Tel.: 212-633-3874, Fax: 212-633-3820, E-mail: reprints@elsevier.com.

Psychiatric Clinics of North America is covered in *MEDLINE/PubMed (Index Medicus)*, *Current Contents/Social and Behavioral Sciences, Social Science Citation Index, Embase/Excerpta Medica,* and PsycINFO.

Contributors

EDITORS

DAN G. BLAZER, MD, MPH, PhD
JP Gibbons Professor Emeritus, Department of Psychiatry and Behavioral Sciences, Professor, Department of Community and Family Medicine, Duke University Medical Center, Durham, North Carolina, USA

SUSAN K. SCHULTZ, MD, DFAPA
Geriatric Psychiatry, James A. Haley Veterans' Hospital, Professor of Psychiatry and Behavioral Neurosciences, University of South Florida, Morsani College of Medicine, Tampa, Florida, USA

AUTHORS

MARILYN ALBERT, PhD
Professor, Department of Neurology, The Johns Hopkins University School of Medicine, Baltimore, Maryland, USA

STEPHEN J. BARTELS, MD, MS
Director, Dartmouth Centers for Health and Aging, Lebanon, New Hampshire, USA

AARTJAN BEEKMAN, MD, PhD
Psychiatrist and Professor, Department of Psychiatry, GGZinGeest and VUmc, Head of the Department of Psychiatry, VUmc University Medical Center Amsterdam Public Health Research Institute, Amsterdam Neuroscience, Amsterdam, The Netherlands

DAN G. BLAZER, MD, MPH, PhD
JP Gibbons Professor Emeritus, Department of Psychiatry and Behavioral Sciences, Professor, Department of Community and Family Medicine, Duke University Medical Center, Durham, North Carolina, USA

CARL I. COHEN, MD
SUNY Distinguished Service Professor and Director, Division of Geriatric Psychiatry, Department of Psychiatry, SUNY Downstate Medical Center, Brooklyn, New York, USA

PETER R. DIMILIA, MPH
Research Assistant, The Dartmouth Institute for Health Policy & Clinical Practice, Lebanon, New Hampshire, USA

ANNEMIEK DOLS, MD, PhD
Psychiatrist and Senior Researcher, Department of Old Age Psychiatry, GGZinGeest and VUmc, Amsterdam Public Health, Amsterdam Neuroscience, Amsterdam, The Netherlands

KAREN L. FORTUNA, PhD
Postdoctoral Fellow, Psychiatry, Geisel School of Medicine at Dartmouth, Hanover, New Hampshire, USA

KSENIA FREEMAN, MD
Department of Psychiatry, SUNY Downstate Medical Center, Brooklyn, New York, USA

LAUREN B. GERLACH, DO
Clinical Lecturer, Program for Positive Aging, Department of Psychiatry, University of Michigan, Ann Arbor, Michigan, USA

BRIAN GHEZELAIAGH, BA
Department of Psychiatry, SUNY Downstate Medical Center, Brooklyn, New York, USA

DINA GHONEIM, MD
Department of Psychiatry, SUNY Downstate Medical Center, Brooklyn, New York, USA

RYAN D. GREENE, Psy D
Department of Psychiatry, Richard L. Roudebush VA Medical Center, Indiana University School of Medicine, Indianapolis, Indiana, USA

TAMMY T. HSHIEH, MD, MPH
Associate Physician, Division of Aging, Department of Medicine, Brigham and Women's Hospital, Instructor in Medicine, Harvard Medical School, Boston, Massachusetts, USA

SHARON K. INOUYE, MD, MPH
Professor of Medicine, Harvard Medical School, Milton and Shirley F. Levy Family Chair, Director, Aging Brain Center, Institute for Aging Research, Hebrew SeniorLife, Boston, Massachusetts, USA

REBEKAH J. JAKEL, MD, PhD
Assistant Professor, Department of Psychiatry and Behavioral Sciences, Duke University Medical Center, Durham, North Carolina, USA

WEI JIANG, MD
Professor, Departments of Psychiatry and Behavioral Sciences and Medicine, Duke University Health System, Durham, North Carolina, USA

HELEN C. KALES, MD
Professor of Psychiatry, Program for Positive Aging, Department of Psychiatry, University of Michigan, Center for Clinical Management Research, VA Ann Arbor Healthcare System, Ann Arbor, Michigan, USA

CHARLES H. KELLNER, MD
Chief of Electroconvulsive Therapy (ECT), New York Community Hospital, Brooklyn, New York, USA

JUSTIN P. MEYER, MD
Assistant Professor, Department of Psychiatry, Icahn School of Medicine at Mount Sinai, New York, New York, USA

JOHN A. NASLUND, PhD, MPH
Research Associate, Center for Technology and Behavioral Health, Lebanon, New Hampshire, USA

ESTHER S. OH, MD, PhD
Associate Professor, Department of Medicine, Division of Geriatric Medicine and Gerontology, The Johns Hopkins University School of Medicine, Baltimore, Maryland, USA

CORINNE PETTIGREW, PhD
Research Associate, Department of Neurology, The Johns Hopkins University School of Medicine, Baltimore, Maryland, USA

KATHERINE RAMOS, PhD
Postdoctoral Fellow, Geriatric, Education, Research and Clinical Center (GRECC), Durham VA Health Care System, Durham, North Carolina, USA

MICHAEL M. REINHARDT, MD
Department of Psychiatry, SUNY Downstate Medical Center, Brooklyn, New York, USA

SUSAN K. SCHULTZ, MD, DFAPA
Geriatric Psychiatry, James A. Haley Veterans' Hospital, Professor of Psychiatry and Behavioral Neurosciences, University of South Florida, Morsani College of Medicine, Tampa, Florida, USA

ANJA SOLDAN, PhD
Assistant Professor, Department of Neurology, The Johns Hopkins University School of Medicine, Baltimore, Maryland, USA

MELINDA A. STANLEY, PhD
Professor, Baylor College of Medicine, Center for Innovations in Quality, Effectiveness and Safety, Michael E. DeBakey VA Medical Center, Houston, Texas, USA

JONATHAN T. STEWART, MD, DFAPA, AGSF
Professor, Psychiatry and Geriatric Medicine, James A. Haley Veterans' Hospital, University of South Florida, College of Medicine, Tampa, Florida, USA

SAMANTHA K. SWETTER, MD
Chief Resident, Department of Psychiatry, Icahn School of Medicine at Mount Sinai, New York, New York, USA

ANINDITHA VENGASSERY, MD
Department of Psychiatry, SUNY Downstate Medical Center, Brooklyn, New York, USA

SOPHIA WANG, MD
Department of Psychiatry, Richard L. Roudebush VA Medical Center, Indiana University School of Medicine, Center of Health Innovation & Implementation Science, Center for Translational Science and Innovation, Sandra Eskenazi Center for Brain Care Innovation, Eskenazi Hospital, Indianapolis, Indiana, USA

Contents

Delirium in the Elderly   1

Tammy T. Hshieh, Sharon K. Inouye, and Esther S. Oh

> Delirium is defined as an acute disturbance in attention and cognition, with significant associated morbidity and mortality. This article discusses the basic epidemiology of delirium and approaches to diagnosing, assessing, and working up patients for delirium. It delineates the pathophysiology and underlying predisposing and precipitating factors for delirium. It also discusses recent advances in prevention and treatment, particularly multicomponent, nonpharmacologic interventions.

Hearing Loss: The Silent Risk for Psychiatric Disorders in Late Life   19

Dan G. Blazer

> Hearing loss is among the most frequent problems experienced by older adults, yet psychiatrists and other clinicians often ignore the problem as an aggravation rather than recognizing that the problem might benefit from appropriate hearing health care. Many psychiatric disorders have been associated with hearing loss, including depression, schizophrenia, and other psychoses, anxiety, and neurocognitive disorders. In this article, hearing loss among older adults is reviewed, with special attention directed toward the recognition and proper referral to a hearing health care provider. Finally, major advances in hearing health care are discussed.

Depression and Cardiovascular Disorders in the Elderly   29

Wei Jiang

> The world's older population continues to grow at an unprecedented rate. This trend amplifies the necessity of improving the care of older patients with chronic health problems. Of those with chronic health problems, those with cardiovascular diseases and depression are particularly challenging due to the multifaceted nature of these conditions. This article discusses the significance of this aging trend and ways to better care for this particular population.

Advances in the Conceptualization and Study of Schizophrenia in Later Life   39

Carl I. Cohen, Ksenia Freeman, Dina Ghoneim, Aninditha Vengassery,
Brian Ghezelaiagh, and Michael M. Reinhardt

> A crisis looms as research and clinical programs have not kept pace with dramatic increases in the number of older adults with schizophrenia. This article provides an overview of the advances in the conceptualization and study of schizophrenia in later life. Theoretic and clinical models in

psychiatry and gerontology are integrated. Specifically, recovery is examined in the context of aging, how clinical dimensionality affects diagnoses in older adults, how various features of schizophrenia are implicated in models of accelerated and paradoxic aging, and how outcome in later life is more dynamic and heterogeneous than assumed previously.

Anxiety disorders in later life are some of the most significant mental health problems affecting older adults. Prevalence estimates of anxiety disorders in late life vary considerably based on multiple methodological issues. Current diagnostic criteria may not adequately capture the nature and experience of anxiety in older people, particularly those in ethnic and racial minority groups. This article reviews late-life anxiety disorders. Pharmacologic and psychotherapy approaches to treat late-life anxiety are reviewed, including a summary of current innovations in clinical care across settings, treatment models, and treatment delivery.

The concept of cognitive reserve (CR) was proposed to account for the discrepancy between levels of brain pathologic features or damage and clinical and cognitive function. This article provides a detailed review of prospective longitudinal studies that have investigated the interaction between CR and Alzheimer disease (AD) biomarkers on clinical and cognitive outcomes among individuals with preclinical AD. Current evidence shows that higher levels of CR are associated with a delay in the onset of symptoms of mild cognitive impairment and that there may be multiple pathways by which CR exerts its protective effects.

Electroconvulsive therapy (ECT) remains an important treatment of geriatric patients. ECT treats severe depression, mania, psychosis, catatonia, and comorbid depression and agitation in dementia. ECT also serves a crucial role in treating urgent illness requiring expedient recovery, such as catatonia, or in patients with severe suicidal ideation or intent. ECT is even more effective in the elderly than in mixed-age adult populations. ECT is a safe treatment option with few medical contraindications. Cognitive effects are largely transient, even in patients with preexisting cognitive impairment.

Further understanding of older age bipolar disorder (OABD) may lead to more specific recommendations for treatment adjusted to the specific characteristics and needs caused by age-related somatic and cognitive changes. Late-onset mania has a broad differential diagnosis and requires full psychiatric and somatic workup, including brain imaging. Research on pharmacotherapy in OABD is limited. First-line treatment of OABD is similar to that for adult bipolar disorder (BD), with specific attention to vulnerability to side effects and somatic comorbidity. Because findings in younger adults with BD cannot be extrapolated to OABD, more research in OABD is warranted.

This article covers current research on the relationship between depression and cognitive impairment in older adults. First, it approaches the clinical assessment of late-life depression and comorbid cognitive impairment. Cognitive risk factors for suicide are discussed. Research is then provided on neuropsychological changes associated with depression, discussing subjective cognitive impairment, mild cognitive impairment, and dementia profiles. In addition, the literature regarding neuroimaging and biomarker findings in depressed older adults is presented. Finally, therapeutic models for the treatment of late-life depression are also discussed, including psychotherapy models, holistic treatments, pharmacologic approaches, and brain-stimulation therapies.

Behavioral and psychological symptoms of dementia (BPSD) are universally experienced by people with dementia throughout the course of the illness and cause a significant negative impact on quality of life for patients and caregivers. Nonpharmacologic treatments have been recommended as first-line treatment of BPSD by multiple professional organizations and should target patients with dementia factors, caregiver factors, and environmental factors. Psychotropic medications are often prescribed off-label without significant evidence to support their use. The Describe, Investigate, Create, Evaluate approach can provide a structured method to investigate and treat BPSD with flexibility to use in multiple treatment settings.

With the growing care needs for the older population at the end of their lives, there has been a substantial increase in attention to the management of the patient with dementia in hospice and palliative care services. This article reviews issues in access to care and the optimal management of the patient with dementia, particularly in the context of neuropsychiatric complexities. Special issues such as delirium, cachexia, behavioral symptoms, and pain management are addressed. Future challenges in research, such as the development of better prognostic models, are noted as well as the importance of attention to access to care.

PSYCHIATRIC CLINICS OF NORTH AMERICA

Preface

Geriatric Psychiatry

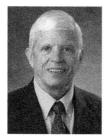 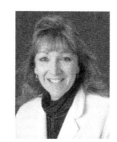

Dan G. Blazer, MD, MPH, PhD   Susan K. Schultz, MD, DFAPA
Editors

The evidence base for treating older adults with psychiatric disorders is ever increasing, yet few persons are trained to treat the elderly through geriatric psychiatry fellowship training programs. Therefore, the bulk of patient care devolves to general psychiatrists, primary care practitioners, and mental health professionals other than psychiatrists. Even so, specialty-trained geriatric psychiatrists must keep up with the latest in our understanding of psychiatric disorders and their comorbidities among older adults. To this end, we have selected an outstanding group of clinicians and clinical investigators to provide an update of a series of topics from which we believe every health care provider for older adults can benefit. Some of the topics are familiar (delirium, depression, and anxiety disorders). Others are less familiar yet most important (psychiatric problems that result from hearing loss, palliative care in dementia and chronic mental illness, and posttraumatic stress disorder [PTSD]).

We begin this issue with an article from Sharon K. Inouye and her colleagues on delirium. They provide a comprehensive review of the epidemiology, etiology, and pathophysiology of delirium. Of most importance, however, they review a nonpharmacologic intervention program that has been demonstrated to be moderately successful in preventing delirium among hospitalized patients. Prevention of delirium may decrease the risk of permanent decline in cognitive function. The article by Dan Blazer reviews the neglected topic by psychiatrists working with the elderly, namely the problems that result from hearing loss and the current treatments for hearing loss about which many psychiatrists are not familiar. Hearing loss is a proven risk for cognitive decline. In the next article, Wei Jiang reviews one of the more frequent, serious, and complex comorbidities faced by clinicians working with older adults: depression and cardiac disorders. Serious cardiac problems increase the risk of depression, and depression increases the risk for adverse outcomes from cardiac problems. The clinician must develop a care plan that combines psychiatric and cardiologic intervention and that complements one another.

Psychiatr Clin N Am 41 (2018) xiii–xv
https://doi.org/10.1016/j.psc.2017.10.014
0193-953X/18/© 2017 Published by Elsevier Inc.

psych.theclinics.com

Schizophrenia is the topic covered in the next article in this issue, where the reader will find an overview of the advances in the conceptualization and study of schizophrenia in later life by Carl I. Cohen and colleagues. In doing this, the authors integrate theoretical and clinical models in psychiatry and gerontology. They examine the concept of recovery from schizophrenia in the context of aging as well as how clinical dimensionality affects diagnoses in older adults. They further address how various features of schizophrenia are implicated in models of accelerated and paradoxical aging, and how outcome in later life is more dynamic and heterogeneous than had been assumed previously. As we experience the aging of our society, including all types of severe mental illness, this article offers new insights on the latest longitudinal findings.

Melinda A. Stanley and her colleague, who have been working for many years in the study of interventions for anxiety disorders in the elderly, review this topic in their article. Anxiety disorders in later life often fly under the radar of health care professionals treating older adults. Though they rarely lead to hospitalization, they are a clear burden for those who suffer, especially when practitioners can do something about them. In the article by Marilyn Albert and her colleagues from Johns Hopkins, an extensive review of cognitive reserve in the elderly is provided. Evidence is mounting that cognitive reserve, as built up over the years via education, participation in cognitive-stimulating activities, and remaining socially engaged, may be one of the more important preventive factors in protecting against the problems that arise from the dementing disorders.

The article by Charles H. Kellner and colleagues addresses an important treatment for geriatric patients, electroconvulsive therapy (ECT). ECT has been long known to provide needed remission of symptoms for older patients with severe depression, mania, psychosis, and catatonia as well as comorbid depression and agitation in dementia. ECT has been shown to be even more effective in the elderly than in mixed-age adult populations. The safety and findings relating to cognition in the context of ECT in older adults are addressed here.

The topic of bipolar disorder occurring in older adults is reviewed comprehensively by Annemiek Dols and Aartjan Beekman. In this article, the condition is termed "older age bipolar disorder" or OABD; the authors describe how a better understanding of late-life symptoms may lead to more specific recommendations for its specific characteristics and needs due to age-related somatic and cognitive changes. The diagnosis of late-onset mania has a broad differential and requires full psychiatric and somatic workup, including brain imaging. First-line treatment is similar as for any adult with bipolar disorder with specific attention to vulnerability to side effects and somatic comorbidity. Future research is needed to clarify best interventions given the limitations in extrapolating data based on younger adults.

In the article by Ryan D. Greene and Sophia Wang in this issue, the authors explore the frequent cooccurrence of depression and neurologic disorders. They emphasize the important yet difficult task of differentiating the symptoms of depression from neurocognitive disorders. Even so, it is critical to make this differentiation so that appropriate therapies can be prescribed.

Behavioral and psychological symptoms of dementia (BPSD) are addressed in the next article by Lauren B. Gerlach and Helen C. Kales. These symptoms are universally experienced in dementia and cause a significant negative impact on quality of life for both patients and caregivers. Nonpharmacologic treatments have been recommended as first-line treatment of BPSD and should target patients with dementia factors, caregiver factors, and environmental factors. The DICE (describe, investigate, create, evaluate) approach can provide a structured method to investigate and treat BPSD with flexibility to use in multiple treatment settings.

The topic of palliative and hospice care is addressed in another article by Jonathan T. Stewart and Susan K. Schultz in this issue. With the growing care needs of the older population at the end of life, there has been a substantial increase in attention to the management of the dementia patient in hospice and palliative care services. This article reviews issues in access to care and the optimal management of the dementia patient particularly in the context of neuropsychiatric complexities. Special issues, such as delirium, cachexia, behavioral symptoms, and pain management, are addressed. Future challenges in research, such as the development of better prognostic models, are noted as well as the importance of attention to access to care.

Stephen J. Bartels and colleagues provide an assessment of opportunities for comprehensive medical and psychiatric care for older persons with chronic mental illness in their article in this issue. They note the important issue that persons with serious mental illness frequently receive inadequate medical care and are more likely to experience difficulty navigating the health care system compared with the general population. Models to address this issue may include programs in collaborative primary care that are designed to create a person-centered care environment for middle-aged and older adults with serious mental illness and medical comorbidity. Peer involvement to engage patient self-management is discussed as an innovative strategy to improve outcomes.

In the article by Rebekah J. Jakel, the rarely discussed yet increasingly important problem of PTSD in later life is explored. We typically associate PTSD with younger persons, often those who have returned from conflicts in Iraq and Afghanistan. Yet PTSD can emerge in later life secondary to service in Vietnam as well as in persons who have experienced other types of traumatic events. PTSD impacts both older men and women.

We planned this issue of *Psychiatric Clinics of North America* so that a range of psychiatric conditions encountered by all health care workers who seek to provide both efficient and effective services to our older citizens would be discussed. Increasing our knowledge is the first step to improving our skills in our mission to this ever-growing segment of our population.

Dan G. Blazer, MD, MPH, PhD
Department of Psychiatry and Behavioral Sciences
Department of Community and Family Medicine
Duke University Medical Center
Box 3
Durham, NC 27710, USA

Susan K. Schultz, MD, DFAPA
Geriatric Psychiatry
James A. Haley Veterans Hospital
University of South Florida
Morsani College of Medicine
13000 Bruce B. Downs Boulevard (116A)
Tampa, FL 33612-4745, USA

E-mail addresses:
dan.g.blazer@duke.edu (D.G. Blazer)
susan-schultz@uiowa.edu (S.K. Schultz)

Delirium in the Elderly

Tammy T. Hshieh, MD, MPH[a],*, Sharon K. Inouye, MD, MPH[b],
Esther S. Oh, MD, PhD[c]

KEYWORDS

- Delirium • Cognitive decline • Dementia • Delirium prevention
- Nonpharmacological interventions

KEY POINTS

- Delirium is a common problem that affects older hospitalized patients, resulting in significant morbidity and mortality.
- Delirium is associated with long-term cognitive and functional decline and is costly to society.
- Delirium is often unrecognized unless actively screened: the Confusion Assessment Method (CAM) provides a simple diagnostic algorithm and is widely used for identification of delirium.
- Delirium is usually due to multifactorial causes and diagnostic evaluation should be targeted based on patient's history and physical examination; cognitive impairment is an important risk factor for delirium.
- Multicomponent, nonpharmacological approaches are the first line of delirium prevention and management strategies.

INTRODUCTION

Delirium is defined as an acute disturbance in attention and cognition that develops over a short period of time. Delirium is the most common complication afflicting hospitalized patients ages 65 years and older, affecting more than 2.6 million older adults each year in the United States.[1] Despite its high prevalence, it often remains unrecognized, with a recent study estimating the rate of undetected delirium to be as high as 60%.[2] Delirium can be a life-threatening condition, yet is often preventable.[1]

Disclosure Statement: The authors have no conflicts of interest and no relationships or financial interests to disclose.
[a] Division of Aging, Department of Medicine, Brigham and Women's Hospital, Harvard Medical School, 1620 Tremont Street, One Brigham Circle, 3rd Floor, Boston, MA 02120, USA; [b] Division of Gerontology, Department of Medicine, Beth Israel Deaconess Medical Center, Harvard Medical School, Aging Brain Center, Institute for Aging Research, Hebrew SeniorLife, 1200 Centre Street, Boston, MA 02131, USA; [c] Division of Geriatric Medicine and Gerontology, Department of Medicine, The Johns Hopkins University School of Medicine, Mason F. Lord Building, 5200 Eastern Avenue, 7th Floor, Room 721, Baltimore, MD 21224, USA
* Corresponding author.
E-mail address: thshieh@bwh.harvard.edu

Psychiatr Clin N Am 41 (2018) 1–17
https://doi.org/10.1016/j.psc.2017.10.001
0193-953X/18/© 2017 Elsevier Inc. All rights reserved.

Hospitalized patients who develop delirium are especially at high risk for long-term cognitive and functional decline. This, in turn, leads to increased posthospitalization treatment costs, including institutionalization, rehabilitation, and home health care services.[1] Total health care costs related to delirium and its complications are estimated at more than $164 billion per year.[3] Because it is highly preventable,[4,5] delirium is increasingly the target for interventions to reduce its associated complications and costs. Nationally, delirium is also considered an important component of patient safety agendas[6] and an important indicator of health care quality of older patients.[7]

EPIDEMIOLOGY

Delirium is often the only sign of a serious underlying medical condition afflicting a patient. **Table 1** demonstrates how common delirium is, with prevalence (present on admission) and incidence (new onset) rates of delirium in various patient populations. The highest incidence rates were observed in the intensive care unit (ICU) and palliative care settings. These rates are likely to be underestimated because many studies of delirium exclude patients with cognitive impairment or dementia at baseline who are particularly vulnerable. The prevalence of delirium in the community is relatively low (1%–2%). This may be because its onset typically brings the patient to emergency care.[1] On presentation to the emergency department, delirium is present in 8% to 17% of older patients and up to 40% of nursing home residents.[1]

Delirium has been consistently associated with poor outcomes, including mortality. Patients with delirium on general medical or geriatric wards are at 1.5-fold increased risk for death in the year following. Delirium in the emergency department is associated with a 70% increased risk of death in the 6 months following the visit.[1,8] Delirium on admission to postacute care is associated with a 5-fold increased risk of 6-month mortality.[9] Delirium in the ICU is associated with a 2-fold to 4-fold increased risk of overall mortality.

Delirium is also associated with long-term cognitive and functional impairment. Delirium in the ICU is associated with cognitive impairment up to 1 year post-discharge.[8] In cardiac surgery patients, a longer duration of delirium ($\geq$3 days) was associated with greater decline in cognitive function after surgery, followed by a slower cognitive recovery over the ensuing 12 months.[10] Physical function is also more significantly impaired after discharge among surgical and nonsurgical patients who develop delirium.[10,11] A recent study showed that delirium was associated with persistent and clinically meaningful impairment of functional recovery up to 18 months later,[12] and that the odds of institutionalization were 2.4-times higher if the patient developed delirium during hospitalization.[13]

DIAGNOSIS, ASSESSMENT, AND WORKUP

The *Diagnostic and Statistical Manual of Mental Disorders*, 5th edition,[14] and the *International Statistical Classification of Diseases and Related Health Problems,* 10th Revision,[15] have specific criteria for delirium that are currently accepted as the diagnostic standard. Expert consensus, however, was used to develop both criteria. The Confusion Assessment Method (CAM)[16] continues to be the most widely used delirium instrument worldwide, used in more than 4500 original studies and translated into more than 20 languages to date. The CAM provides an algorithm based on the 4 core features of delirium: acute onset, fluctuating course of symptoms, inattention, and either disorganized thinking or altered level of consciousness.[17] The CAM algorithm has been validated in high-quality studies and has high sensitivity (94%–100%) and specificity (90%–95%)

Table 1
Incidence of delirium and associated outcomes, by population

	Prevalence (%)[a]	Incidence (%)[a]	Outcomes (Adjusted RR[b])
Surgical			
Cardiac	—	11–46	Cognitive dysfunction 1.7; functional decline 1.9
Non-cardiac	—	13–50	Functional decline 2.1; cognitive dysfunction 1.6
Orthopaedic	17	12–51	Dementia or cognitive dysfunction 6.4–41.2; admission to institution 5.6
Medical			
General medical	18–35	11–14	Mortality 1.5–1.6; functional decline 1.5
Old age medicine	25	20–29	Falls 1.3; mortality 1.9; admission to institution 2.5
Intensive care	7–50	19–82	Mortality 1.4–13.0; longer length of stay 1.4–2.1; extended mechanical ventilation 8.6
Stroke	—	10–27	Mortality 2.0; any of increased length of stay, functional impairment, or death 2.1
Dementia	18	56	Cognitive decline 1.6–3.1; admission to an institution 9.3; mortality 5.4
Palliative care, cancer	—	47	—
Nursing home or postacute care	14	20–22	Mortality 4.9
Emergency department	8–17	—	Mortality 1.7

Some data are provided as ranges. All values were derived from selected articles with sample sizes of 100 or more that satisfied the Strengthening the Reporting of OBservational studies in Epidemiology (STROBE) criteria for setting, participants, measurement, and statistical methods, and included a validated delirium instrument. An additional inclusion criterion for incidence studies was serial delirium assessments no more than 3 days apart by trained research staff or clinicians. The appendix contains a complete list of references and further details on all articles.

Abbreviation: RR, relative risk.

[a] Sum of prevalence and incidence yields overall occurrence rates of delirium in each setting.

[b] Derived from studies that provided adjustment for at least one covariable.

Reprinted from The Lancet, Volume 383, No. 9920. Inouye SK, Westendorp RG, Saczynski JS. Delirium in elderly people. Pages 911-922, Copyright 2014, with permission from Elsevier.

with high interrater reliability.[18] The CAM has also been adapted for use in the ICU,[19] emergency departments,[20] nursing homes, and palliative care; it is included as part of the Minimum Data Set.[21] Since the development of the CAM tool almost 3 decades ago, more than 25 other delirium screening tools have been developed.[22] A brief assessment for the CAM is the 3 minute-diagnostic assessment (3D)-CAM, which provides an assessment in a 20-item checklist that streamlines evaluation of the 4 CAM features, with sensitivity of 95% and specificity of 94% in hospitalized patients.[23] Another brief test is the 4A's Test (4AT), which has been validated in clinical settings involving dementia patients and is easy to administer, with a sensitivity of 90% and specificity of 84%.[24]

Behavioral checklists for symptoms of delirium have also been developed, particularly for nursing-based studies, including the Delirium Observation Screening Scale,[25] the Nursing Delirium Screening Checklist,[26] and the Neelon and Champagne (NEE-CHAM) Confusion Scale.[27] Delirium severity has become increasingly important because it can assist with tracking the clinical course and response to treatment within a delirium episode. Some of the more widely used delirium severity measurement tools include the Delirium Rating Scale-Revised-98 (DRS-R-98)[28] and the Memorial Delirium Assessment Scale (MDAS).[29] Another delirium severity assessment tool is the CAM-Severity (CAM-S) scale, which was developed based on the CAM.[18] It has strong neuropsychological properties and high predictive validity for clinical outcomes, including length of stay, hospital costs, institutionalization, and mortality.[18] The previously mentioned Delirium Observation Screening Scale, a nursing-administered tool that can be used to assess delirium severity, has been found to correlate strongly with the Delirium Rating Scale.[30]

A validated chart review-based method for identifying delirium has been developed[31]; however, its sensitivity is limited compared with interview-based methods. Combining chart review with direct patient interviews captures the highest number of patients with delirium and maximizes sensitivity for delirium detection.[32] The Family CAM (FAM-CAM) has also been developed as a validated way of determining delirium based on reports by informal caregivers.[33]

Delirium is missed by clinicians in up to 70% of delirious patients.[34] Because of its fluctuating nature and varying behavioral presentations (ie, hypoactive, hyperactive, and mixed), detecting and studying delirium can be challenging. Clinically, it requires insightful judgment and thorough medical evaluation. In research and quality improvement, the combined method of interview plus chart review is likely the highest-yield approach.[32] Once suspected, the clinician should assess for recent changes in medications, new infections, or recent medical illnesses that may be contributing. Acute onset, fluctuations and changes in attention are central features of delirium. Therefore, it is important to establish a patient's baseline cognitive function. Detailed background interview with a proxy informant, such as a family member, caregiver, or medical professional who knows the patient, is essential in determining the change in a patient's mental status.

The cognitive evaluation for delirium should include global cognitive changes, impairment in attention, disorganized thought processes, and altered level of consciousness. Global cognitive changes can be assessed through simple cognitive testing, combined with close clinical observations of behavior, such as the patient's ease and fluidity, and ability to stay on tasks. Brief cognitive screening should involve formal cognitive tests, such as the Short Portable Mental Status Questionnaire,[35] Mini-Cog,[36] or Montreal Cognitive Assessment.[37] Inattention, a hallmark feature of delirium, is clinically manifested by difficulties in focusing on the task at hand, maintaining a conversation, and/or shifting of attention. Disorganized thought is present when the patient's speech is incoherent, rambling, or lacks logical presentation of ideas. Altered consciousness can be highly variable and range from agitation to lethargy or stupor. Other clinical features that are commonly associated with delirium but that are not diagnostic criteria include psychomotor agitation, paranoid delusions, sleep-wake cycle disruption, and emotional lability. If time is extremely limited, a 2-item questionnaire with "months of the year backwards" and "what is the day of the week?" has been shown to have sensitivity of 93% and specificity of 64% for identifying delirium.[38]

Clinically, delirium typically presents as hypoactive, hyperactive, or mixed behavior. The hypoactive form is characterized by lethargy and reduced psychomotor function. It is associated with poorer prognosis, possibly in part because it is more often unrecognized by clinicians and caregivers.[34] The reduced level of patient activity in hypoactive delirium is often misattributed to low mood or fatigue. The hyperactive form of delirium is rarely unnoticed and characterized by agitation, increased vigilance, and sometimes, hallucinations. In the mixed form of delirium, patients fluctuate between the hypoactive and the hyperactive forms. The mixed form of delirium can be challenging to diagnose because patients fluctuate between hypoactivity and hyperactivity.

Table 2 proposes a suggested work-up for delirium. Of note, delirium may be the initial or only sign of a serious and life-threatening underlying illness, such as sepsis, pneumonia, or myocardial infarction. Further complicating the evaluation is the frequently atypical presentations of disease in older persons. Diagnostic evaluation for delirium should be targeted based on the patient's history and physical examination because unfocused testing is likely to result in low diagnostic yield.[39]

It is also important to differentiate delirium from dementia or recognize when delirium is superimposed on dementia. Delirium superimposed on dementia results in worsened cognitive and functional decline, increased hospital length of stay, increased

Table 2
Assessment of suspected delirium

Assessment	Actions
History	Check baseline cognitive function and recent (within past 2 weeks) changes in mental status (eg, family, staff)
	Recent changes in disorder, new diagnoses, complete review of systems
	Review all current drugs (including over-the-counter and herbal preparations); pay special attention to new drugs and drug interactions
	Review alcohol and sedative use
	Assess for pain and discomfort (eg, urinary retention, constipation, thirst)
Vital signs	Measure temperature, oxygen saturation, fingerstick glucose concentration
	Take postural vital signs as needed
Physical and neurological examination	Search for signs of occult infection, dehydration, acute abdominal pain, deep vein thrombosis, other acute illness; assess for sensory impairments
	Search for focal neurological changes and meningeal signs
Targeted laboratory assessment (selected tests based on clues from history and physical)[a]	Consider full blood count; urinalysis; measurement of concentrations of electrolyres, calcium, and glucose; measurement of renal, liver, and thyroid function; taking cultures of urine, blood, sputum; measurement of drug concentrations; measurement of concentrations of ammonia, vitamin B12, and cortisol
	Measure arterial blood gas
	Do electrocardiography
	Chest radiography
	Lumbar puncture should be reserved for assessment of fever with headache and meningeal signs or suspicion of encephalitis
Targeted neuroimaging (selected patients)	Assess focal neurological changes (stroke can present as delirium)
	Test for suspected encephalitis (for temporal lobe changes)
	Assess patients with histories or signs of head trauma
Electroencephalography (selected patients)	Assess for occult seizures
	Differentiate psychiatric disorder from delirium

[a] Not all of these tests should be done in all patients; rather, specific tests should be guided by history, physical examination, and previous results.

Reprinted from The Lancet, Volume 383, No. 9920. Inouye SK, Westendorp RG, Saczynski JS. Delirium in elderly people. Pages 911-922, Copyright 2014, with permission from Elsevier.

readmission rates, institutionalization, and death.[40–43] The key diagnostic feature that helps differentiate the 2 conditions is the acute and rapid onset of delirium with its hallmark of inattention, whereas dementia is more gradual. Establishing the occurrence of acute change can be difficult if no baseline cognitive data are available, preexisting cognitive deficits are not clearly reported by an informant, or patients are uncooperative.

Delirium should also be differentiated from psychiatric conditions such as depression, mania, and schizophrenia. In general, these conditions do not develop suddenly when a patient is acutely ill, hospitalized, or undergoing surgery. Given the seriousness of delirium and that certain medical treatments may actually worsen symptoms, it is best to manage these patients as cases of delirium until further diagnostic information is available.

The electroencephalogram (EEG) has limited utility in the diagnosis of delirium. Delirium severity does result in a characteristic diffuse slowing, poor organization of background rhythm, and increased theta and delta activity. The current role for EEG is in differentiating delirium from other causes in patients who are difficult to assess.[44] EEG can be particularly useful in patients with dementia who develop acute mental status changes and to identify occult seizures (eg, nonconvulsive status epilepticus, focal dyscognitive seizures, or atypical complex partial seizures).[44–46]

No specific laboratory tests currently exist that will definitively determine the diagnosis of delirium. Laboratory tests for delirium are intended for identifying potential contributing factors to address and are guided by astute clinical judgment. Evaluation for occult infection and other laboratory tests should be considered as indicated by history, physical examination, and preliminary laboratory findings, including chest radiograph, blood cultures, urinalysis, thyroid function, arterial blood gas, vitamin B-12 level, cortisol level, electrocardiogram, and toxicology screen.

In general, routine request of neuroimaging studies for delirium is not recommended because the overall diagnostic yield is low. In fact, neuroimaging changes the management of patients in less than 10% of cases.[47] Brain imaging is recommended in cases of head trauma, new focal neurologic symptoms, suspected encephalitis, or fever of unknown origin.[48] Lumbar puncture should be considered in cases in which suspicion of meningitis, encephalitis, or vasculitis must be ruled out.[49]

PATHOPHYSIOLOGY OF DELIRIUM

The fundamental pathophysiological mechanisms underlying delirium remain unclear. Increasing evidence suggests that multiple biological factors interact and result in disruption of large-scale neuronal networks in the brain, leading to acute confusion, cognitive dysfunction, and delirium.[50] **Table 3** explores potential pathophysiological pathways underlying delirium.

Although many different neurotransmitters and biomarkers are implicated in delirium (see **Table 3**), among the most frequently considered mechanisms of delirium is cholinergic dysfunction. Acetylcholine plays a key role in mediating consciousness and attentional processes, and thus may contribute to the acute confusional state, often with alterations of consciousness, seen with delirium. Evidence for the cholinergic hypothesis include findings that anticholinergic drugs can induce delirium in humans and animals and that serum anticholinergic activity is increased in patients with delirium.[51,52] However, at this time, there is no clear evidence that cholinesterase inhibitors prevent incident delirium.[53]

Chronic stress induced by severe illness, trauma, or surgery often activates the sympathetic and immune systems and may contribute to delirium. This activation may involve hypercortisolism, altered thyroid function, modified blood-brain barrier permeability, and release of cerebral cytokines that alter neurotransmitter function.[54] Because inflammation is considered to play an important role in the pathogenesis of delirium,[55] much

Table 3
Potential pathophysiological contributors to delirium

	Type of data available	Review published
Neurotransmitters		
Acetylcholine	Experimental and observational	Yes
Dopamine	Experimental and observational	Yes
γ-aminobutyric acid	Experimental and observational	No
Melatonin	Experimental and observational	Yes
Tryptophan or serotonin	Observational	Yes
Glutamate	Observational	No
Epinephrine or norepinephrine	Hypothetical	No
Proinflammatory markers		No
Interferon α or β	Experimental	Yes
Interleukin 6	Observational	Yes
Interleukin 8	Observational	Yes
Interleukin 10	Observational	No
Tumour necrosis factor α	Hypothetical	Yes
Interleukin 1β	Hypothetical	Yes
Prostaglandin E	Hypothetical	Yes
Physiological stressors		No
Cortisol	Observational	No
S100β	Observational	No
Neopterin	Observational	No
Hypoxia	Observational	No
Metabolic disorders		No
Lactic acidosis	Experimental and observational	No
Hypoglycaemia or hyperglycaemia	Observational	No
IGF1	Observational	Yes
Hypercapnia	Hypothetical	Yes
Electrolyte disorders		No
Sodium, calcium, magnesium	Experimental and observational	No
Genetic factors		
Apolipoprotein E	Observational	Yes
Glucocorticoid receptor	Observational	No
Dopamine transporter or receptor	Observational	Yes
Toll-like receptor 4	Hypothetical	No

Experimental means that controlled data—eg, from clinical trials or inference from unintended side-effects in human beings, or both—are available. Observational means that only observational data are available in human beings. Hypothetical means that that studies in human beings are not yet available to support the mechanism.
    Reprinted from The Lancet, Volume 383, No. 9920. Inouye SK, Westendorp RG, Saczynski JS. Delirium in elderly people. Pages 911-922, Copyright 2014, with permission from Elsevier.

attention has been focused on inflammatory biomarkers for identifying patients at higher risk for delirium and elucidating the underlying pathophysiology of delirium. Recent studies on interleukins and C-reactive protein have shown that they may be promising as biomarkers of delirium in the future.[56,57] However, no biomarkers under investigation are currently validated or available for clinical diagnosis or monitoring of delirium.

Neuroimaging studies, using either computed tomography or MRI, have demonstrated structural abnormalities in the brains of patients with delirium. Regions of particular interest include the splenium of the corpus callosum, thalamus, and right temporal lobe.[58–62] Advanced neuroimaging techniques have found global and regional perfusion abnormalities in delirious patients.[63,64] Functional imaging may help determine structural damage resulting from an episode of delirium.[65] Most recently, studies in surgical patients have found that microstructural changes in the limbic and memory structures of the brain, plus structural dysconnectivity involving interhemispheric and fronto-thalamic-cerebellar networks, may predispose patients to delirium.[66]

RISK FACTORS FOR DELIRIUM: PREDISPOSING AND PRECIPITATING

Delirium is commonly multifactorial in older persons, although a single factor can precipitate delirium.[67] The development of delirium typically involves complex interrelationships between multiple predisposing factors that make a patient more vulnerable to insults and the degree of exposure to noxious insults or precipitating factors. For example, a single low dose of sedative (eg, benzodiazepine) given to a patient who is cognitively impaired may lead to delirium. However, a patient without severe illness or cognitive impairment may be able to withstand repeated exposures to multiple insults such as surgery, anesthesia, and hospitalization, as well as sedative or other medications, before developing delirium.[68] Addressing only a single noxious insult is likely insufficient in preventing or improving delirium. Rather, multicomponent approaches are recommended for both prevention and treatment.[69,70]

Table 4 presents predisposing and precipitating factors identified in previous, validated studies. The leading risk factors consistently identified in both medical and noncardiac surgery populations are dementia or cognitive impairment, functional impairment, vision impairment, history of alcohol abuse, and advanced age (>70 years). Comorbidity burden or the presence of specific comorbidities, such as stroke and depression, was associated with an increased risk for delirium in all patient populations. ICU studies usually included younger patients and, therefore, baseline factors (eg, dementia, functional impairment) were not significant predictors of delirium. Precipitating factors varied more across patient populations. In medical patients, polypharmacy, psychoactive medication use, and physical restraints were the leading factors, conferring up to a 4.5-fold increased risk. Abnormal laboratory values increased risk by 40% to 50% in all populations.

ADVANCES IN PREVENTION AND TREATMENT

Recent systematic reviews and guidelines have presented an evidence-based approach to delirium prevention and management. In 2014, the American Geriatrics Society and the American College of Surgeons jointly released clinical practice guidelines for postoperative delirium prevention and treatment.[71] These guidelines underscore the importance of nonpharmacologic multicomponent prevention strategies, ongoing education of health care providers, medical workup for the cause of delirium, optimizing pain control with nonopioids, and avoiding high-risk medications (**Box 1**). The guidelines also recommended against treating hypoactive delirium pharmacologically and against using benzodiazepines, except in alcohol or benzodiazepine withdrawal-related delirium.

Nonpharmacological Prevention and Management

Preventing delirium before it develops is the most effective strategy against complications associated with delirium (**Table 5**). The Hospital Elder Life Program (HELP) uses a multicomponent intervention in preventing delirium and is the

Table 4
Risk factors for delirium from validated predictive models

	General Medicine	Surgery Non-cardiac	Cardiac	Intensive-Care Unit
Predisposing factors				
Dementia	2.3–4.7	2.8	—	—
Cognitive impairment	2.1–2.8	3.5–4.2	1.3	—
History of delirium	—	3.0	—	—
Functional impairment	4.0	2.5–3.5	—	—
Visual impairment	2.1–3.5	1.1–3.0	—	—
Hearing impairment	—	1.3	—	—
Comorbidity or severity of illness	1.3–5.6	4.3	—	1.1
Depression	3.2	—	1.2	—
History of transient ischaemia or stroke	—	—	1.6	—
Alcohol misuse	5.7	1.4–3.3	—	—
Older age (≥75 y)	4.0	3.3–6.6	—	1.1
Precipitating factors				
Drugs				
Several drugs used	2.9	—	—	—
Psychoactive drugs	4.5	—	—	—
Sedatives or hypnotics	—	—	—	4.5
Use of physical restraints	3.2–4.4	—	—	—
Use of bladder catheter	2.4	—	—	—
Physiological				
Increased serum urea	5.1	—	—	1.1
Increased BUN:creatinine ratio	2.0	2.9	—	—
Abnormal serum albumin	—	—	1.4	—
Abnormal sodium, glucose, or potassium	—	3.4	—	—
Metabolic acidosis	—	—	—	1.4
Infection	—	—	—	3.1
Any iatrogenic event	1.9	—	—	—
Surgery				
Aortic aneurysm	—	8.3	—	—
Non-cardiac thoracic	—	3.5	—	—
Neurosurgery	—	—	—	4.5
Trauma admission	—	—	—	3.4
Urgent admission	—	—	—	1.5
Coma	—	—	—	1.8–21.3

Data are relative risks. Some data are reported as ranges.
Abbreviation: BUN, blood urea nitrogen.
Reprinted from The Lancet, Volume 383, No. 9920. Inouye SK, Westendorp RG, Saczynski JS. Delirium in elderly people. Pages 911-922, Copyright 2014, with permission from Elsevier.

Box 1
Drugs to use with caution in delirium: summary of Beers criteria (2015)

Anticholinergics
  Antihistamines (including first-generation)
  Antiparkinson agents
  Skeletal muscle relaxants
  Antidepressants (particularly amitriptyline, desipramine, doxepin, nortriptyline, paroxetine)
  Antipsychotics
  Antimuscarinics
  Antispasmodics
  Antiemetics

All antipsychotics

Benzodiazepines (short, intermediate, and long-acting)

Chlorpromazine

Corticosteroids

H2-receptor antagonists
  Cimetidine
  Famotidine
  Nizatidine
  Ranitidine

Meperidine

Sedative hypnotics

Adapted from American Geriatrics Society 2015 Beers Criteria Update Expert Panel. American Geriatrics Society 2015 updated beers criteria for potentially inappropriate medication use in older adults. J Am Geriatr Soc 2015;63(11):2231-43.

---

most widely disseminated approach.[67] In a recent meta-analysis of 14 interventional studies based on HELP, multicomponent nonpharmacological approaches significantly reduced the incidence of delirium and falls among older hospitalized, non-ICU patients.[70] Effective nonpharmacological treatment approaches include reorientation (eg, using orientation boards, calendars, clocks), hydration, sleep enhancement, therapeutic activities, encouraging the presence of family members, and private rooms closer to the nurses' station for increased supervision. Sensory deficits should be assessed and corrected by ensuring that all assistive devices such as eyeglasses and hearing aides are readily available and properly used. Physical restraints should be minimized due to their role in prolonging delirium, worsening agitation, and increasing risk of strangulation.[72] Strategies that increase the patient's mobility, self-care, and independence should be routinely reinforced. A recent Cochrane review of delirium prevention examined 39 trials involving 16,092 subjects and found moderate quality evidence that multicomponent nonpharmacologic interventions are effective for delirium prevention but less robust for decreasing delirium severity or duration.[53]

Geriatric assessment followed by consultation has also been successful in preventing and treating delirium, although the impact depends on adherence of the staff to recommendations made by the geriatric consultants.[1,5] The consultative strategy focused on the specific domains of adequate brain oxygen delivery, fluid and electrolyte balance, pain management, reduction in psychoactive medications, bowel and bladder function, nutrition, early mobilization, prevention of postoperative complications, appropriate environmental stimuli, and treatment of delirium. Controlled trials of educational strategies targeted toward health care staff and tailoring multifactorial treatments to individual

Table 5 Management of suspected delirium	
Management	**Actions**
Drug adjustments	Reduce or remove psychoactive drugs (eg, anticholinergics, sedatives or hypnotics, opioids); lower dosages; avoid as required dosing Substitute less toxic alternatives Use non-pharmacological approaches for sleep and anxiety, including music, massage, relaxation techniques
Address acute medical issues	Treat problems identified in work-up (eg, infection, metabolic disorders) Maintain hydration and nutrition Treat hypoxia
Reorientation strategies	Encourage family involvement; use companions as needed Address sensory impairment; provide eyeglasses, hearing aids, interpreters
Maintain safe mobility	Avoid use of physical restraints, tethers, and bed alarms Ambulate patient at least three times per day; active range-of-motion Encourage self-care and regular communication
Normalise sleep–wake cycle	Discourage napping and encourage exposure to bright light during the day Try to provide uninterrupted period for sleep at night Provide non-pharmacological sleep protocol and quiet room at night with low level lighting
Pharmacological management	Reserve for patients with severe agitation that interrupts essential treatment (eg, intubation) or severe psychotic symptoms Start with low doses and titrate until effect achieved; haloperidol 0.25–0.5 mg orally or intramuscularly twice a day is preferred; atypical antipsychotics close in effectiveness

Reprinted from The Lancet, Volume 383, No. 9920. Inouye SK, Westendorp RG, Saczynski JS. Delirium in elderly people. Pages 911-922, Copyright 2014, with permission from Elsevier.

needs have demonstrated improved recognition and reduced incidence and/or duration of delirium.[73–76] Other effective approaches include interventions delivered by family members, and mobility or rehabilitation interventions.[77–79]

One recent pilot study examined modified HELP in long-term care for prevention and treatment of delirium and found it was feasible, with high satisfaction rates and decreased hospitalization.[80] A recent clinical trial using daily therapeutic activities that stimulate cognition in the postacute care setting for delirium superimposed on dementia found no impact on delirium duration or severity but did demonstrate significant improvement in executive function and decreased length of stay.[81] Other studies have focused on specialized delirium rooms, geriatric units, music therapy, and improving sleep, with varying results.[82–84]

Pharmacologic Prevention and Management

Although clinical trials have used a variety of pharmacologic approaches, there is no convincing evidence that these treatments are effective for prevention or treatment of delirium. Most published pharmacologic trials report no difference in delirium rates or duration.[1] In a recent Cochrane review examining antipsychotic medications for preventing delirium in hospitalized non-ICU subjects, there was no clear benefit in using antipsychotics.[53] On meta-analysis, the review also found minimal evidence to support the use of other medications such as cholinesterase inhibitors, melatonin, and melatonin-receptor agonists (ramelteon) in preventing delirium.[53] In trials that did find reduced delirium following targeted pharmacologic treatment, there was no improvement in clinical outcomes, such as ICU or hospital length of stay, hospital complications, or mortality. A recent systematic review examined antipsychotic drugs risperidone, olanzapine, quetiapine, ziprasidone, and haloperidol.[85] It found no significant decrease in delirium incidence among 19 studies, and no change in delirium duration or severity, hospital or intensive care length of stay, or mortality.[85] Potential harm was demonstrated in 3 studies in which more subjects required institutionalization after treatment with antipsychotics. In a recent randomized controlled trial of atypical antipsychotic drugs in palliative care, participants receiving oral risperidone or haloperidol had higher delirium symptom scores and worse overall survival.[86] Perioperatively, no measures, including different types of sedation and anesthesia, have shown benefit in decreasing delirium incidence. It remains unclear if dexmedetomidine is effective, even in subpopulations of patients with cognitive impairment.[87] Adjusting the depth of anesthesia according to bispectral index monitoring may decrease the incidence of delirium.[53] Given the evidence, pharmacologic prevention and treatment are not recommended at this time. We recommend reserving the use of antipsychotics and other sedating medications for treatment of severe agitation that poses risk to safety.[69,85,88]

CHALLENGES AND SUMMARY

Delirium remains a common and morbid condition for older adults who can be highly vulnerable to this multifactorial syndrome. Prevention with multicomponent nonpharmacological approaches remains important. Treatment, however, has been challenging and many treatments have their own risks and costs for the individual patient. In the future, approaches to preventing and treating delirium will need to be streamlined to recruit multiple types of caregivers and health care providers. Thus, the wave of the future may be to develop pathophysiologically targeted approaches to diagnosis and treatment to move the field ahead.

REFERENCES

1. Inouye S, Westendrop R, Saczynski J. Delirium in elderly people. Lancet 2014; 383(9920):911–22.
2. de la Cruz M, Fan J, Yennu S, et al. The frequency of missed delirium in patients referred to palliative care in comprehensive cancer center. Support Care Cancer 2015;23(8):2427–33.
3. Leslie D, Marcantonio E, Zhang Y, et al. One-year health care costs associated with delirium in the elderly population. Arch Intern Med 2008;168(1):27–32.
4. Inouye SK, Bogardus ST Jr, Charpentier PA, et al. A multicomponent intervention to prevent delirium in hospitalized older patients. N Engl J Med 1999;340(9): 669–76.
5. Marcantonio ER, Flacker JM, Wright RJ, et al. Reducing delirium after hip fracture: a randomized trial. J Am Geriatr Soc 2001;49(5):516–22.
6. Wachter R. Understanding patient safety. New York: McGraw Hill Medical; 2012.
7. National Quality Measures. Delirium: proportion of patients meeting diagnostic criteria on the Confusion Assessment Method (CAM). 2003;2017(05/26). Available at: https://www.qualitymeasures.ahrq.gov/summaries/summary/27635?. Accessed November 23, 2017.
8. Pandharipande PP, Girard TD, Jackson JC, et al. Long-term cognitive impairment after critical illness. N Engl J Med 2013;369(14):1306–16.
9. Marcantonio ER, Kiely DK, Simon SE, et al. Outcomes of older people admitted to postacute facilities with delirium. J Am Geriatr Soc 2005;53(6):963–9.

10. Saczynski JS, Marcantonio ER, Quach L, et al. Cognitive trajectories after post-operative delirium. N Engl J Med 2012;367(1):30–9.
11. Rudolph JL, Jones RN, Levkoff SE, et al. Derivation and validation of a preoperative prediction rule for delirium after cardiac surgery. Circulation 2009;119(2): 229–36.
12. Hshieh TT, Saczynski J, Gou RY, et al. Trajectory of functional recovery after post-operative delirium in elective surgery. Ann Surg 2017;265(4):647–53.
13. Witlox J, Eurelings LS, de Jonghe JF, et al. Delirium in elderly patients and the risk of postdischarge mortality, institutionalization, and dementia: a meta-analysis. JAMA 2010;304(4):443–51.
14. American Psychiatric Association, editor. Diagnostic and statistical manual of mental disorders. Washington, DC: American Psychiatric Society; 2013.
15. World Health Organization. The ICD-10 classification of mental and behavioural disorders: diagnostic criteria for research. Geneva (Switzerland): World Health Organization; 1993.
16. Inouye SK, van Dyck CH, Alessi CA, et al. Clarifying confusion: the confusion assessment method: a new method for detection of delirium. Ann Intern Med 1990;113(12):941–8.
17. Wei L, Fearing M, Sternberg E, et al. The Confusion Assessment Method: a systematic review of current usage. J Am Geriatr Soc 2008;56(5):823–30.
18. Inouye SK, Kosar CM, Tommet D, et al. The CAM-S: development and validation of a new scoring system for delirium severity in 2 cohorts. Ann Intern Med 2014; 160(8):526–33.
19. Ely EW, Margolin R, Francis J, et al. Evaluation of delirium in critically ill patients: validation of the Confusion Assessment Method for the Intensive Care Unit (CAM-ICU). Crit Care Med 2001;29(7):1370–9.
20. Han JH, Zimmerman EE, Cutler N, et al. Delirium in older emergency department patients: recognition, risk factors, and psychomotor subtypes. Acad Emerg Med 2009;16(3):193–200.
21. Centers for Medicare and Medicaid Services. Minimum data set, version 3.0. Washington, DC: Centers for Medicare and Medicaid Services; 2010.
22. De J, Wand A. Delirium screening: a systematic review of delirium screening tools in hospitalized patients. Gerontologist 2015;55(6):1079–99.
23. Marcantonio E, Ngo L, O'Connor M, et al. 3D-CAM: derivation and validation of a 3-minute diagnostic interview for CAM-defined delirium: a cross-sectional diagnostic test study. Ann Intern Med 2014;161(8):554–61.
24. Bellelli G, Morandi A, Davis D, et al. Validation of the 4AT, a new instrument for rapid delirium screening: a study in 234 hospitalised older people. Age Ageing 2014;43(4):496–502.
25. Schuurmans MJ, Shortridge-Baggett LM, Duursma SA. The delirium observation screening scale: a screening instrument for delirium. Res Theory Nurs Pract 2003;17(1):31–50.
26. Gaudreau J, Gagnon P, Harel F, et al. Fast, systematic, and continuous delirium assessment in hospitalized patients: the nursing delirium screening scale. J Pain Symptom Manage 2005;29(4):368–75.
27. Neelon VJ, Champagne MT, Carlson JR, et al. The NEECHAM Confusion Scale: construction, validation, and clinical testing. Nurs Res 1996;45(6):324–30.
28. Trzepacz PT, Mittal D, Torres R, et al. Validation of the Delirium Rating Scale-revised-98: comparison with the delirium rating scale and the cognitive test for delirium. J Neuropsychiatry Clin Neurosci 2001;13(2):229–42.

29. Breitbart W, Rosenfeld B, Roth A, et al. The memorial delirium assessment scale. J Pain Symptom Manage 1997;13(3):128–37.
30. Scheffer A, van Munster B, Schuurmans M, et al. Assessing severity of delirium by the delirium observation screening scale. Int J Geriatr Psychiatry 2011; 26(3):284–91.
31. Inouye SK, Leo-Summers L, Zhang Y, et al. A chart-based method for identification of delirium: validation compared with interviewer ratings using the Confusion Assessment Method. J Am Geriatr Soc 2005;53(2):312–8.
32. Saczynski JS, Kosar CM, Xu G, et al. A tale of two methods: chart and interview methods for identifying delirium. J Am Geriatr Soc 2014;62(3):518–24.
33. Steis MR, Evans L, Hirschman KB, et al. Screening for delirium using family caregivers: convergent validity of the family confusion assessment method and interviewer-rated Confusion Assessment Method. J Am Geriatr Soc 2012; 60(11):2121–6.
34. Inouye SK, Foreman MD, Mion LC, et al. Nurses' recognition of delirium and its symptoms: comparison of nurse and researcher ratings. Arch Intern Med 2001; 161(20):2467–73.
35. Pfeiffer E. A short portable mental status questionnaire for the assessment of organic brain deficit in elderly patients. J Am Geriatr Soc 1975;23(10): 433–41.
36. Borson S, Scanlan J, Benedict L, et al. The mini-cog: a cognitive 'vital signs' measure for dementia screening in multi-lingual elderly. Int J Geriatr Psychiatry 2000; 15(11):1108–13.
37. Nasreddine ZS, Phillips NA, Bédirian V, et al. The Montreal Cognitive Assessment, MoCA: a brief screening tool for mild cognitive impairment. J Am Geriatr Soc 2005;53(4):695–9.
38. Fick DM, Inouye SK, Guess J, et al. Preliminary development of an ultrabrief two-item bedside test for delirium. J Hosp Med 2015;10(10):645–50.
39. Hirano LA, Bogardus ST, Saluja S, et al. Clinical yield of computed tomography brain scans in older general medical patients. J Am Geriatr Soc 2006;54(4): 587–92.
40. Jackson JC, Gordon SM, Hart RP, et al. The association between delirium and cognitive decline: a review of the empirical literature. Neuropsychol Rev 2004; 14(2):87–98.
41. Gross A, Jones R, Habtemariam D, et al. Delirium and long-term cognitive trajectory among persons with dementia. Arch Intern Med 2012;172(17):1324–31.
42. Fick D, Steis M, Waller J, et al. Delirium superimposed on dementia is associated with prolonged length of stay and poor outcomes in hospitalized older adults. J Hosp Med 2013;8(9):500–5.
43. Morandi A, Davis D, Fick D, et al. Delirium superimposed on dementia strongly predicts worse outcomes in older rehabilitation in patients. J Am Med Dir Assoc 2014;15(5):349–54.
44. Sutter R, Ruegg S, Tschudin-Sutter S. Seizures as adverse events of antibiotic drugs: a systematic review. Neurology 2015;85(15):1332–41.
45. Jenssen S. Electroencephalogram in the dementia workup. Am J Alzheimers Dis Other Demen 2005;20(3):159–66.
46. Tu T, Loh N, Tan N. Clinical risk factors for non-convulsive status epilepticus during emergent electroencephalogram. Seizure 2013;22(9):794–7.
47. Hirao K, Ohnishi T, Matsuda H, et al. Functional interactions between entorhinal cortex and posterior cingulate cortex at the very early stage of Alzheimer's

disease using brain perfusion single-photon emission computed tomography. Nucl Med Commun 2006;27(2):151–6.

48. Lai M, Wong TND. Intracranial cause of delirium: computed tomography yield and predictive factors. Intern Med J 2012;42(4):422–7.

49. Marcantonio E. In the clinic. Delirium. Ann Intern Med 2011;154(11):ITC6-1. ITC6-16.

50. Watt D, Budding D, Koziol L. Delirium and confusional states. In: Noggle C, Dean R, editors. Disorders in neuropsychiatry. New York: Springer; 2013. p. 425–40.

51. Hshieh TT, Fong TG, Marcantonio ER, et al. Cholinergic deficiency hypothesis in delirium: a synthesis of current evidence. J Gerontol A Biol Sci Med Sci 2008; 63(7):764–72.

52. Lauretani F, Ceda GP, Maggio M, et al. Capturing side-effect of medication to identify persons at risk of delirium. Aging Clin Exp Res 2010;22(5–6):456–8.

53. Siddiqi N, Harrison J, Clegg A, et al. Interventions for preventing delirium in hospitalised non-ICU patients. Cochrane Database Syst Rev 2016;(3):CD005563.

54. Hughes CG, Patel MB, Pandharipande PP. Pathophysiology of acute brain dysfunction: what's the cause of all this confusion? Curr Opin Crit Care 2012; 18(5):518–26.

55. MacLullich AM, Ferguson KJ, Miller T, et al. Unravelling the pathophysiology of delirium: a focus on the role of aberrant stress responses. J Psychosom Res 2008;65(3):229–38.

56. Vasunilashorn S, Ngo L, Inouye S, et al. Cytokines and postoperative delirium in older patients undergoing major elective surgery. J Gerontol A Biol Sci Med Sci 2015;70(10):1289–95.

57. Dillon S, Vasunilashorn S, Ngo L, et al. Higher C-reactive protein levels predict postoperative delirium in older patients undergoing major elective surgery: a longitudinal nested case-control study. Biol Psychiatry 2017;81(2):145–53.

58. Bogousslavsky J, Ferrazzini M, Regli F, et al. Manic delirium and frontal-like syndrome with paramedian infarction of the right thalamus. J Neurol Neurosurg Psychiatr 1988;51(1):116–9.

59. Doherty MJ, Jayadev S, Watson NF, et al. Clinical implications of splenium magnetic resonance imaging signal changes. Arch Neurol 2005;62(3):433–7.

60. Naughton BJ, Moran M, Ghaly Y, et al. Computed tomography scanning and delirium in elder patients. Acad Emerg Med 1997;4(12):1107–10.

61. Ogasawara K, Komoribayashi N, Kobayashi M, et al. Neural damage caused by cerebral hyperperfusion after arterial bypass surgery in a patient with moyamoya disease: case report. Neurosurgery 2005;56(6):E1380.

62. Takanashi J, Barkovich AJ, Shiihara T, et al. Widening spectrum of a reversible splenial lesion with transiently reduced diffusion. AJNR Am J Neuroradiol 2006; 27(4):836–8.

63. Fong TG, Bogardus ST Jr, Daftary A, et al. Cerebral perfusion changes in older delirious patients using 99mTc HMPAO SPECT. J Gerontol A Biol Sci Med Sci 2006;61(12):1294–9.

64. Pfister D, Siegemund M, Dell-Kuster S, et al. Cerebral perfusion in sepsis-associated delirium. Crit Care 2008;12(3):R63.

65. Choi S, Lee H, Chung T, et al. Neural network functional connectivity during and after an episode of delirium. Am J Psychiatry 2012;169(5):498–507.

66. Cavallari M, Dai W, Guttmann C, et al. Neural substrates of vulnerability to post-surgical delirium as revealed by presurgical diffusion MRI. Brain 2016;139(Pt 4): 1282–94.

67. Inouye SK, Charpentier PA. Precipitating factors for delirium in hospitalized elderly persons: predictive model and interrelationship with baseline vulnerability. JAMA 1996;275(11):852–7.
68. Gleason OC. Donepezil for postoperative delirium. Psychosomatics 2003;44(5): 437–8.
69. O'mahony R, Murthy L, Akunne A, et al. Synopsis of the National Institute for Health and Clinical Excellence guideline for prevention of delirium. Ann Intern Med 2011;154(11):746–51.
70. Hshieh T, Yue J, Oh E, et al. Effectiveness of multicomponent nonpharmacological delirium interventions: a meta-analysis. JAMA Intern Med 2015;175(4):512–20.
71. American Geriatrics Society Expert Panel on Postoperative Delirium in Older Adults. American Geriatrics Society abstracted clinical practice guideline for postoperative delirium in older adults. J Am Geriatr Soc 2015;63(1):142–50.
72. Inouye SK, Zhang Y, Jones RN, et al. Risk factors for delirium at discharge: development and validation of a predictive model. Arch Intern Med 2007;167(13):1406–13.
73. Marcantonio ER, Bergmann MA, Kiely DK, et al. Randomized trial of a delirium abatement program for postacute skilled nursing facilities. J Am Geriatr Soc 2010;58(6):1019–26.
74. Deschodt M, Braes T, Flamaing J, et al. Preventing delirium in older adults with recent hip fracture through multidisciplinary geriatric consultation. J Am Geriatr Soc 2012;60(4):733–9.
75. Lundström M, Edlund A, Karlsson S, et al. A multifactorial intervention program reduces the duration of delirium, length of hospitalization, and mortality in delirious patients. J Am Geriatr Soc 2005;53(4):622–8.
76. Pitkala KH, Laurila JV, Strandberg TE, et al. Multicomponent geriatric intervention for elderly inpatients with delirium: a randomized, controlled trial. J Gerontol A Biol Sci Med Sci 2006;61(2):176–81.
77. Caplan GA, Coconis J, Board N, et al. Does home treatment affect delirium? A randomised controlled trial of rehabilitation of elderly and care at home or usual treatment (The REACH-OUT trial). Age Ageing 2006;35(1):53–60.
78. Martinez FT, Tobar C, Beddings CI, et al. Preventing delirium in an acute hospital using a non-pharmacological intervention. Age Ageing 2012;41(5):629–34.
79. Schweickert WD, Pohlman MC, Pohlman AS, et al. Early physical and occupational therapy in mechanically ventilated, critically ill patients: a randomised controlled trial. Lancet 2009;373(9678):1874–82.
80. Boockvar K, Teresi J, Inouye S. Preliminary Data: An Adapted Hospital Elder Life Program to Prevent Delirium and Reduce Complications of Acute Illness in Long-Term Care Delivered by Certified Nursing Assistants. J Am Geriatr Soc 2016; 64(5):1108–13.
81. Kolanowski A, Fick D, Litaker M, et al. Effect of cognitively-stimulating activities on symptom management of delirium superimposed on dementia: a randomized controlled trial. J Am Geriatr Soc 2016;64(12):2424–32.
82. Flaherty J, Little M. Matching the environment to patients with delirium: lessons learned from the delirium room, a restraint-free environment for older hospitalized adults with delirium. J Am Geriatr Soc 2011;59(s2):S295–300.
83. Van Rompaey B, Elseviers M, Van Drom W, et al. The effect of earplugs during the night on the onset of delirium and sleep perception: a randomized controlled trial in intensive care patients. Crit Care 2012;16(3):1–10.
84. Yang J, Choi W, Ko Y, et al. Bright light therapy as an adjunctive treatment with risperidone in patients with delirium: a randomized, open, parallel group study. Gen Hosp Psychiatry 2012;34(5):546–51.

85. Neufeld K, Yue J, Robinson T, et al. Antipsychotic medication for prevention and treatment of delirium in hospitalized adults: a systematic review and meta-analysis. J Am Geriatr Soc 2016;64(4):705–14.

86. Agar MR, Lawlor PG, Quinn S, et al. Efficacy of oral risperidone, haloperidol, or placebo for symptoms of delirium among patients in palliative care: a randomized clinical trial. JAMA Intern Med 2017;177(1):34–42.

87. Liu Y, Ma L, Gao M, et al. Dexmedetomidine reduces postoperative delirium after joint replacement in elderly patients with mild cognitive impairment. Aging Clin Exp Res 2016;28(4):729–36.

88. Barr J, Fraser GL, Puntillo K, et al. Clinical practice guidelines for the management of pain, agitation, and delirium in adult patients in the intensive care unit. Crit Care Med 2013;41(1):263–306.

Hearing Loss

The Silent Risk for Psychiatric Disorders in Late Life

Dan G. Blazer, MD, MPH, PhD

KEYWORDS

- Hearing loss • Schizophrenia • Depression • Hearing aids • Red flag conditions
- Ototoxicity • Neurocognitive disorders

KEY POINTS

- Hearing loss is a silent epidemic among older adults. Nearly 30 million Americans experience hearing loss, and the prevalence increases dramatically with age.
- Hearing loss is associated with many psychiatric disorders, including depression, anxiety, schizophrenia and other psychoses, and cognitive impairment.
- Psychiatrists are in an excellent position to identify hearing loss given that when they administer a mental status examination the older adult may expose the disorder through answers that suggest the question was misunderstood.
- Knowing the services available to those with hearing loss is key to a proper referral and follow-up of older adults identified as experiencing the problem.

INTRODUCTION

Hearing loss in later life is among the most common impairments experienced and among the most easily underdiagnosed and unappreciated in terms of the potential for significant risk of both physical and psychiatric problems.[1] The loss can be gradual or acute (usually gradual for older adults) and can lead to problems with communication, quality of life issues such as increased isolation, and significant financial challenges. Despite the problems associated with hearing loss, many older adults do not seek hearing health care, and when they do, they find the care to not be optimal. A pair of hearing aids (which are not covered by Medicare) cost on average around $4700, including professional services.[1(p207)] In addition, these devices are often not deemed useful to older adults once purchased, so they are relegated to a bureau drawer.

Disclosures: The author chaired the National Academies Committee on Accessible and Affordable Hearing Health Care for Adults (2016). No other disclosures.
JP Gibbons Professor Emeritus of Psychiatry and Behavioral Sciences, Duke University Medical Center, Box 3003, 3521 Hosp South, Durham, NC 27710, USA
E-mail address: dan.g.blazer@dm.duke.edu

Psychiatr Clin N Am 41 (2018) 19–27
https://doi.org/10.1016/j.psc.2017.10.002

A most understudied area is the risk for psychiatric disorders and emotional stress related to hearing loss. This article provides some background into the world of hearing loss and hearing health care providers, the current literature on the association of hearing loss and psychiatric disorders, the expanded horizons of assistance provided for hearing health care, and the role of geriatric mental health care workers in assuring the best possible treatment for hearing problems in older adults (**Table 1**).

EPIDEMIOLOGY OF HEARING LOSS IN LATER LIFE

Determining the prevalence of hearing loss must not be based solely upon self-report. The Centers for Disease Control and Prevention (CDC) report that 1 in 4 US adults who report excellent-to-good hearing already experience hearing damage.[3] Prevalence and incidence studies typically measure severity by the decibels (dB) that can be

Table 1 Definitions	
Deaf	A community and culture of individuals with shared language (American Sign Language) and cultural values and priorities. The deaf are not discussed in this article.
Hearing Loss	Hearing function that is poorer than normal in the general population and applied to persons who were not born with hearing impairment. Loss usually begins in middle or late life and progresses over the years. It can range from difficulty in hearing quiet sounds such as a whisper to profound loss that totally eliminates effective communication except through adaptations such as lip reading.[1]
Hearing Health Care	All forms of care provided to persons with hearing loss ranging from devices for individuals such as hearing aids and training by audiologists in practices to improve comprehension to environmental provisions (such as loop technology, which connects hearing aids with microphones in an auditorium).[1] When hearing loss is profound and cannot be corrected, cochlear implants are a last resort approach to care and can be remarkably effective.
Otolaryngologists	Physicians trained in ear, nose and throat conditions. They roughly can be divided into those who focus on hearing loss, including surgery, treatment of infections of the ear, removal of cerumen, as well as inserting cochlear implants, and those who engage in other disorders (such as tumors of the head and neck). About 10,000 practice in the United States.[1]
Audiologist	Nonphysician health care professionals trained in the assessment treatment and prevention of hearing, balance, and related disorders. They usually have attained a doctoral degree in audiology and are licensed by states. Around 12, 250 audiologists practice in the United States.[1]
Hearing Instrument Specialists	Individuals trained to identify individuals with hearing loss, fit individuals with hearing aids, and educate persons and their families who experience hearing loss. Relatively short training period followed by an internship. Licensed by states. About 5570 practice in the United States.[1]
Red Flag Conditions	Several conditions are signals of serious or readily treatable causes of hearing loss according to the FDA. These include: active drainage from the ear, sudden-onset or rapidly progressing hearing loss, acute or chronic dizziness, sudden or rapidly progressive hearing loss in 1 ear, visible evidence of significant cerumen within the ear canal, and pain or discomfort in the ear.[2]

heard. For all ages, the normal person can hear sounds at less than 26 dB. Persons with mild hearing loss can hear sounds between 26 to 40 dB; those with moderate loss hear 41 to 70 dB, and those with severe loss hear 71 or more dB. The prevalence of hearing loss of mild-to-severe loss in the Framingham Heart Study was 29% for subjects 63 to 95 years.[3] National Health and Nutrition Examination Survey (NHANES) investigators found the frequency in men 70 years of age and older to be 44.8%.[1(p43)] In the Health ABC study (ages 73–84), 76.9% of subjects were found to have loss of hearing for high-frequency sounds (inability to hear higher frequency sounds is more prevalent than for low frequency sounds in older adults). Hearing loss is typically greater for men than for women over age 70.[4] In the Framingham study the incidence of hearing loss was 8.4% in the right ear and 13.7% in the left ear over a 6-year follow-up of persons 58 to 86 years of age.[1(p46)]

In the NHANES study, investigators found a lower prevalence of hearing loss among African Americans compared with non-Hispanic whites. Prevalence for Mexican Americans was approximately equal to that among whites.[5] Hearing loss for all older adults appears to be declining as younger birth cohorts are experiencing a lower rate of loss than older cohorts, although as noted previously, it remains a major impairment.[5] This trend is surprising given the exposure to loud sounds via smartphones and ear buds. As would be expected, with aging, the onset and progression of hearing loss increase, in 1 study by 0.7 to 1.2 dB per year. In summary, hearing loss progresses gradually over time, although it accelerates among the oldest old.

Risk factors for hearing loss in later life include lower socioeconomic status, a long history of smoking, higher systolic blood pressure, obesity, high waist circumference, highly elevated glycosylated hemoglobin, atherosclerosis, and many ototoxic medications such as nonsteroidal anti-inflammatory drugs (NSAIDs) and acetaminophen. One area that is receiving increased attention is noise-induced hearing loss. The CDC[3] recently issued a report suggestion that 1 in 2 US adults with hearing damage from noise did not have noisy jobs, and the resulting problems with hearing derive from noise exposure such as using a leaf blower, attending a sporting event, or being close to a siren for an extended period of time. They determined that noises above 85 dB can cause hearing damage.

PSYCHIATRIC DISORDERS SECONDARY TO HEARING LOSS

To gain a perspective on psychiatric problems associated with hearing loss, the clinician must have an appreciation of the problems faced by those with the impairment. Persons with hearing loss have difficulty following a conversation if there is background noise, such as in a restaurant. They become frustrated when trying to communicate with their families. Although they can hear speech, that speech may be muffled, because they can understand only portions of the conversation. This problem can be partially corrected if they can see the person talking and learn to read lips. In addition, the standard treatment is hearing aids, yet these aids are expensive and often not as effective as desired, leading to more frustration. Clinicians should also recognize that hearing loss in older adults will be more likely hidden from clinicians and family. Elders may even become more adaptable to the impairment than young adults. For example, in 1 study, younger adults reported being lonely at a higher frequency than older adults with hearing loss.[6]

The association of hearing loss with paranoid disorders has long been investigated by psychiatrists, yet the empirical evidence is mixed. For example, Kay and Roth explored whether deafness, along with abnormalities of personality and loss of many relatives, contributed to more social isolation in a paraphrenic population of older adults than in mood disorder patients. (Paraphrenia was a term used frequently by psychiatrists decades ago to describe older patients who developed delusions and occasionally hallucinations without the loss of intellect or personality.) They found some impairment in hearing in 40% of the British paraphrenic patients; in 15% of patients, it was of marked degree. In Sweden, only the most severe cases of hearing loss had been recorded, and the prevalence was 16% among paraphrenics. The frequency of hearing loss in patients with affective disorders was only 7%. Although associated with the prevalence of paraphenia, visual or hearing loss did not seem to modify the symptomatology of paraphrenia greatly.[7] Felix Post, in a report from 1966, found that among 72 patients with paranoid disorder, 25% experienced hearing loss compared with 11% of controls.[8] Since these early publications, the belief has been prevalent among psychiatrists that hearing loss is associated with paranoid psychoses, although this has not much been explored during the past few years in the psychiatric literature.

In a more recent meta-analysis of epidemiologic studies, the investigators found an increased risk of hearing impairment for all psychosis outcomes, such as hallucinations, delusions, psychotic symptoms, and delirium, although the odds ratios were relatively small. Early exposure to hearing impairment led to elevated the risk of later development of schizophrenia. The investigators suggested that potential mechanisms underlying this association include loneliness and disturbances of source monitoring (locating the source of sounds and interpreting these sounds).[9]

In another study, self-reported hearing impairment was associated with increased frequency of psychotic symptoms among those using a hearing aid in younger persons but not older adults.[10] Following up this study, the same team found that although social isolation and loneliness were both associated with psychosis, perhaps related to an inability to interpret the environment in which they lived, the level of complexity of the social world in urban settings compared with rural settings explained most of the individual's inability to correctly process this information and therefore increased the likelihood of psychosis.[11]

Other psychiatric symptoms are also associated with hearing loss, especially depression and anxiety. Thomas and colleagues[12] found a fourfold increase in scores above a clinically significant cutoff for anxiety and depression symptoms among patients with a hearing impairment compared with the general population. In another study among community respondents in underserved areas and using self-rated scales, subjects who reported sensory loss had high rates of depression and a compromised quality of life compared with respondents without these impairments.[13] In yet another study, investigators explored the associated relationship of hearing impairment with anxiety symptoms. They found that, compared with individuals with no hearing impairment, the odds of prevalent anxiety were significantly higher among individuals with mild hearing impairment, and for those with moderate or severe impairment the odds were even greater. Hearing aid use was not significantly associated with lower likelihood of anxiety.[14] Not all studies, however, confirm the association of hearing loss with psychiatric disorders, especially for major depression.[15]

Recent attention has been directed toward the risk for cognitive decline secondary to hearing loss. Findings from a chart review of 133 patients 50 years of age and older suggest that hearing loss is highly prevalent among this sample of cognitively impaired older adults. Sixty percent of the sample had at least a mild hearing loss in the better hearing ear. Among variables examined, age and medical history of diabetes were also strongly associated with hearing impairment. Hearing aid utilization increased with the severity of hearing loss, from 9% to 54% of individuals with a mild or moderate/severe hearing loss, respectively. No evidence was available, however, as to whether the use of hearing aids improved or slowed the decline in cognition.[16] In a more refined study, consistent peripheral hearing was significantly related to 10 of 11 measures of cognition that assessed processing speed, executive function, or memory, as well as global cognitive status.[17]

The Treatment of Hearing Loss

The recognition and treatment of hearing loss should be the responsibility of all health care professionals working with older adults. From the perspective of the psychiatrist and other mental health care workers, referring their patients to the appropriate specialists along with a discussion as to the significant risks of leaving hearing loss unattended is the most important point. To engage older patients and their families about hearing loss and its treatment, the mental health care worker must have a working knowledge of the hearing health care workforce and the services that can be offered.

Four disciplines should be at the front line.[1(pp76,77)] Audiologists are trained in assessment and treatment, including the dispensing of hearing aids as well as rehabilitation of hearing loss and related problems (such as problems with balance and tinnitus). Hearing instrument specialists are qualified to identify individuals with hearing loss (through basic audiologic testing), dispense and adjust hearing aids, and educate clients and family members about hearing loss. A small fraction of otolaryngologists dispense hearing aids yet are key in treating the red flag conditions noted previously as well as inserting cochlear implants. The practitioners from each of these 3 disciplines tend to cluster in large metropolitan areas.

As can be recognized from the small number of persons specializing in hearing health care, the burden of identifying and referring individuals for hearing health care among the professions usually falls to primary care physicians (including geriatricians) and other specialties, perhaps especially psychiatrists. Primary care physicians are in the best position to identify hearing loss among older adults, such as during the annual wellness visit under Medicare, yet many elders do not take advantage of this visit. Given the busy practices of primary care doctors, checking for hearing loss, even via a simple question such as "Are you having any trouble with your hearing?" is limited, especially since checking for hearing loss is not a required screen as set up by the US Preventive Services Task Force for adults 50 years of age and older.[18] In addition, the quiet physician's office where the older adult is usually face-to-face with the doctor is not ideal for determining the degree of impairment that is present.

Psychiatrists and other mental health workers, when they suspect hearing loss in their patients, are in an excellent position to determine if hearing loss is present. Responses to questions to test cognitive function may be inaccurate in part because the questions are misunderstood or not answered. Other queries frequently are misinterpreted. Patients may complain that they forgot their hearing aid or they place the aid in their ear during the session. In addition, the older adult is often accompanied by a family member who can inform the psychiatrist about hearing loss. Final determination of the extent of hearing loss should be delegated to an audiologist who can perform appropriate testing. Formal screening by the audiologist (including the audiogram) is covered by Medicare if referred by a physician, an option all too often a neglected. However, audiologists are not reimbursed for any treatment of the problem such as rehabilitation and fitting of hearing aids.

The physician should also determine if the older adult is taking a potentially ototoxic medication. The most common of these are: aspirin, NSAIDs, some antibiotics, diuretics such as furosemide and bumetanide, and some anticancer drugs. Hearing loss has been rarely reported for some psychotropic drugs such as olanzapine, carbamazepine, and valproic acid. Some selective serotonin reuptake inhibitors can cause tinnitus.[19] If tinnitus is a major concern, patients may be switched to mirtazapine, which has not been found to cause tinnitus. Almost all older persons have lost hearing in the higher frequencies and frequencies below 25 dB. Therefore, the speech frequency range that renders understanding of soft speech in a quiet room difficult is a frequent problem for older adults.[20] It usually occurs gradually and bilaterally, because of changes in the inner ear.

All clinicians should be aware of more serious and/or treatable causes of hearing loss among older adult, the most common being cerumen impaction (unilateral or bilateral), which can be treated by an audiologist, otolaryngologist, or even self-removal with ceruminolytics or irrigation. Other red flag conditions listed by the US Food and Drug Administration (FDA) and requiring referral to a physician with experience in treating hearing problems have already been noted.[21] Unilateral hearing loss is a potentially serious condition that should lead to an immediate referral to an otolaryngologist, because it may be the primary symptom of an acoustic neuroma or a cholesteatoma.

Once referred to a hearing health care specialist for treatment, several options are available to persons with hearing loss. Hearing aids are the standard treatment and what most consumers consider initially as the first-line treatment. Yet hearing aids are expensive, costing around $4700 for a pair of medium range aids in the United States in 2013, this cost including both the hearing aid itself and the services of the audiologist or hearing instrument specialist.[22] Therefore cost is an initial barrier to hearing aid use. Yet for those who have purchased hearing aids, they frequently are not used following initial adjustments. Primary reasons for nonuse are perception that the hearing aids are not effective, difficulty fitting (adjustment of the hearing aid to the proper pitch and frequency), maintenance (such as changing batteries), stigma, and ongoing costs of batteries, maintenance, and repair. Frustration with hearing aids may lead individuals to decide that they can manage without the hearing aid.[23] In a sample of the patients aged 50 years and older from the NHANES, 3.8 million Americans wore hearing aids, but only 14.2% with hearing loss used hearing aids.[24]

Yet for many, hearing aids significantly reduce the impairment that results from hearing loss. In 1 study, the use of hearing aids was associated with improved minimental state performance.[25,26] This suggested to the authors that hearing loss was associated with sensory specific cognitive decline rather than global cognitive impairment.

Recently, bipartisan legislation was introduced by Senators Elizabeth Warren (D-Mass) and Chuck Grassley (R-Iowa) to permit the sale of over-the-counter hearing aids.[27] These devices will not replace clinician-prescribed hearing aids but are focused upon improving hearing for those with mild-to-moderate impairment. There would be some FDA regulation, but that regulation would be minimal yet protect against problems such as sound intensity being set dangerously high. Therefore, cost should significantly be reduced, and persons who believe they might benefit from such an instrument would be much more willing to expend a few hundred dollars rather than thousands. Personal sound amplification products (PSAPs) are already widely available, advertised frequently in the media, yet they cannot be recommended as a hearing aid at present. Many people, however, do purchase them, and some may even today meet the standards for an over-the-counter device.

Several other hearing assistive technologies are available. These include hearing induction loop and telecoil technologies that allow the sound system in a room to connect wirelessly with an individual's hearing via a telecoil in the hearing aid and the installation of hearing loop wiring around the perimeter of the room that connects to the room's sound system (ideal for group gatherings where speakers use microphones such as worship services). This combination can reduce background noise and improve the clarity of sound.[1(p162)] Another option, although less frequently used, is captioning of a talk or conversation using transcription (similar to that used by court reporting and projected onto a screen in the room). Yet another approach is the production of apps for smart phones, which in combination with Bluetooth technology, can permit, for example, placing a smart phone in the center of the table of a noisy restaurant and using an earpiece connected to the device to amplify the conversation at the table.

Treatment of hearing loss does not stop with technological assistance. Auditory rehabilitation is an evidenced-based intervention.[28] These programs are designed to help individuals learn to adapt to their hearing loss, become familiar with hearing-assistive technologies, learn strategies for better listening and communication, and provide psychosocial support.[1(p86–88)] The programs can be group based or individualized. Audiologists and speech and language pathologists can administer these programs.

SUMMARY

In general, hearing health care technology is at a point where a combination of opening the market to new products coupled with new and disruptive technologies may significantly change the options persons with hearing loss have available as well as decrease the stigma of seeking and using hearing assistive technologies and approaches to rehabilitation. Psychiatrists and other mental health professionals should be aware of this changing landscape and take advantage of their unique opportunity to recognize hearing loss and refer their patients to professionals or even to the local drug store to seek products that can assist them to hear better. Data are not yet available that definitively demonstrate improved hearing can reduce the frequency of psychiatric disorders including cognitive impairment. Yet there is reason to believe that improved hearing will at least improve the quality of life of those experiencing such loss.

REFERENCES

1. National Academies of Science. Engineering and medicine: hearing health care for adults: priorities for improving access and affordability. Washington, DC: The National Academies Press; 2016.
2. Federal Drug Administration. Red Flag Conditions Available at: https://ihsinfo.org/IhsV2/hearing_professional/2003/010_January-February/030_FDA_Red_Flags.cfm. Accessed March 1, 2017.
3. Centers for Disease Control and Prevention. Vital signs: too loud! For too long! Loud noises damage hearing. 2017. Available at: www.cdc.gov/vitalsigns/HearingLoss. Accessed April 26, 2017.
4. Cruickshanks KJ, Wiley TL, Tweed TS, et al. The 5-year incidence and progression of hearing loss: the epidemiology of hearing-loss study. Arch Otolaryngol Head Neck Surg 2003;129:1041–6.
5. Gates GA, Cooper JC Jr, Kannel WE, et al. Hearing in the elderly: the Framingham cohort, 1983-1985. Part I. Basic audiometric test results. Ear Hear 1990; 11:247–56.
6. Sung YK, Li L, Blake C, et al. Association of hearing loss and loneliness in older adults. J Aging Health 2016;28:979–94.

7. Kay DW, Roth R. Environmental and hereditary factors in the schizophrenias of old age ("late paraphrenia") and their bearing on the general problem of causation in schizophrenia. J Ment Sci 1961;107:649–86.
8. Post F. Persistent persecutory states of the elderly. Oxford (England): Pergamon Press; 1966.
9. Linszen MM, Brouwer RM, Heringa SM, et al. Increased risk of psychosis in patients with hearing impairment: review and meta-analyses. Neurosci Biobehav Rev 2016;62:1–20.
10. van der Werf M, van Boxtel M, Verhey F, et al. Mild hearing impairment and psychotic experiences in a normal aging population. Schizophr Res 2007;94:180–6.
11. van der Werf M, van Winkel R, van Boxtel M, et al. Evidence that the impact of hearing impairment on psychosis risk is moderated by the level of complexity of the social environment. Schizophr Res 2010;122:193–8.
12. Thomas A. Acquired hearing loss: psychological and social implications. Orlando (FL): Academic Press; 1984.
13. Armstrong TW, Surya S, Elliott TR, et al. Depression and health-related quality of life among persons with sensory disabilities in a health professional shortage area. Rehabil Psychol 2016;61:240–50.
14. Contrera KJ, Betz J, Deal J, et al, Health ABC Study. Association of hearing impairment and anxiety in older adults. J Aging Health 2016;29:172–84.
15. Mener DJ, Betz J, Genther DJ, et al. Hearing loss and depression in older adults. J Am Geriatr Soc 2013;61:1627–9.
16. Nirmalasari O, Mamo SK, Nieman CL, et al. Age-related hearing loss in older adults with cognitive impairment. Int Psychogeriatr 2017;29:115–21.
17. Harrison Bush AL, Lister JJ, Lin FR, et al. Peripheral hearing and cognition: evidence from the staying keen in later life (SKILL) study. Ear Hear 2015;36: 395–407.
18. Available at: https://www.uspreventiveservicestaskforce.org/Page/Document/UpdateSummaryFinal/hearing-loss-in-older-adults-screening. Accessed March 22, 2017.
19. Cianfrone G, Pentangelo D, Cianfrone E, et al. Pharmacological drugs inducing ototoxicity, vestibular symptoms and tinnitus: a reasoned and updated guide. Eur Rev Med Pharmacol Sci 2011;15:601–36.
20. Available at: https://www.nidcd.nih.gov/health/age-related-hearing-loss#1. Accessed March 22, 2017.
21. Available at: https://www.slideshare.net/HISDepartment/fda-regulations-for-hearing-instrument-specialists. Accessed March 22, 2017.
22. Strom K. HR 2013 hearing aid dispenser survey. Available at: http://www.hearingreview.com/2014/04/hr-2013-hearing-aid-dispenser-survey-dispensing-age-internet-big-box-retailers-comparison-present-past-key-business-indicators-dispensing-offices/. Accessed March 22, 2017.
23. McCormack A, Fortnum H. Why do people fitted with hearing aids not wear them. Int J Audiol 2013;52:360–8.
24. Chien W, Lin FR. Presence of hearing aid use among older adults in the United States. Arch Intern Med 2012;172:292–3.
25. Qian ZJ, Wattamwar K, Caruana FF, et al. Hearing aid use is associated with better mini-mental state exam performance. Am J Geriatr Psychiatry 2016;24: 694–702.
26. Folstein MF, Folstein SE, McHugh PR. "Mini-Mental State." A practical method for grading the cognitive state of patients for the clinician. J Psychiatr Res 1975;12: 189–98.

27. Warren E, Grassley C. Over-the-counter hearing aids: the path forward. JAMA Intern Med 2017;177(5):609–10.

28. Chisolm T, Arnold M. Evidence about the effectiveness of aural rehabilitation programs for adults. In: Wong L, Hickson L, editors. Evidence-based practice in audiology: evaluating interventions for children and adults with hearing impairment. San Diego (CA): Plural Publishing; 2012. p. 237–66.

Depression and Cardiovascular Disorders in the Elderly

Wei Jiang, MD[a,b],*

KEYWORDS

- Elderly • Depression • Cardiovascular disease • Prevalence • Mechanisms
- Intervention

KEY POINTS

- Both depression and cardiovascular diseases are highly prevalent in elder individuals.
- Depression and cardiovascular diseases have a synergetic impact on prognosis of elder patients and they share similar pathologic mechanisms.
- Prompt recognition of depression in patients with cardiovascular disease is necessary.
- Applying evidence-based intervention that targets depression in elderly patients, especially those with cardiovascular diseases, will improve the outcomes of these patients.

The world's older population continues to grow at an unprecedented rate. Currently, 8.5% of people worldwide (617 million) are 65 years and older and this percentage is projected to jump to nearly 17% of the world's population by 2050 (1.6 billion).[1] Cardiovascular disease (CVD) and depression are among the most common diseases experienced by this older population. According to the statistics of *Aging in the United States* (2016),[2] the present population of 46 million Americans aged 65 years and older is projected to more than double to more than 98 million by 2050, and this group's share of the total population will increase to nearly 24% from 15%. This trend amplifies the necessity of improving care for older patients with chronic health problems. Of those with chronic health problems, those with CVD and depression are particularly challenging due to the multifaceted nature of these conditions. This review focuses on the significance of this aging trend and ways to better care for this particular population.

Disclosure Statement: The author does not have any financial relationship with any companies.
[a] Department of Psychiatry and Behavioral Sciences, Duke University Health System, Durham, NC 27710, USA; [b] Department of Medicine, Duke University Health System, Durham, NC 27710, USA
* 1108 Grogans Mill Drive, Cary, NC 27519.
E-mail address: jiang001@mc.duke.edu

Psychiatr Clin N Am 41 (2018) 29–37
https://doi.org/10.1016/j.psc.2017.10.003
0193-953X/18/© 2017 Elsevier Inc. All rights reserved.

psych.theclinics.com

THE SIGNIFICANCE OF DEPRESSION AND CARDIOVASCULAR DISEASE IN THE ELDERLY

The growing population of elderly is a sign of success reflecting several merits in societal enhancement. However, although people are living longer, they are increasingly battling chronic diseases of the heart, respiratory system, and the brain. With the growth of the younger population slowing, meeting the demand of the health care needs of the elderly has emerged as a significant public health burden for prevention and treatment. Of these chronic diseases, CVD has been the largest global disease burden in people aged 60 years and older, occupying about one-third of the total global disease burden.[3] An estimated 85.6 million of American adults (>1 in 3) have 1 or more types of CVD. Of these, more than a half (43.7 million) of are estimated to be 60 years of age or older. The prevalence of CVD is positively related to age. For instance, in the age group from 60 to 79 years old, 69.1% of men and 67.9% of women experience CVD; in the 80 years and older group, 84.7% of men and 85.9% of women have CVD. The leading causes of death in men and women 65 years of age or older are diseases of the heart.[4] Elderly patients with CVD account for more than 65% of the total spending of US CVD patients on personal health care and public health.[5]

Mental health concerns are also age-related issues. It is estimated that 20% of people aged 55 years or older experience some type of mental health concern,[6] with the most common conditions being anxiety, severe cognitive impairment, and depression. Depression affects approximately 20 million Americans every year, regardless of age, race, or gender. Depression in the elderly is generally considered to be 2 types: late-onset that develops when an individual reaches 60 years or older, and younger onset that persists into late life.[7] Recognizing certain features of these 2 kinds of depression can be helpful when developing appropriate care plans (**Table 1**). Although depression is not a normal part of the aging process, there is a strong likelihood of it occurring when other physical health conditions are present. For example, nearly one-fourth of the 600,000 people who experienced a stroke in a given year experienced clinical depression.[8] Differing rates of depression in the elderly have been reported due to variations in study designs, including the population studied, study size, tools of assessments, and so forth.

Table 1
Features differ between and early-onset and late-onset of depression

Features of Depression	Early-Onset	Late-Onset
Genetic	Higher with more family history of mental illnesses	Low
Risk factors	Higher rate of personality disorders	Higher rate of CVD risk factors
Brain abnormality	Functional	Structural
Cognitive or neurologic	Fewer issues	More issues
Depression manifestation	Expressive depressive symptoms	Somatic and cognitive
Obtain psychiatric care	More likely to need formal mental health care	Generally not recognized until late
Comorbidities	Greater substance abuse and dependence	Greater physical comorbidities
Suicide	At risk for suicide	Highest risk of suicide
Response to depression intervention	More responsive	More resistant

Studies investigating whether the prevalence of depression is more or less common in the elderly compared with younger individuals have generally shown younger adults to have a higher frequency of depression. The prevalence of past-year mood, anxiety, and substance use disorders, as well as lifetime personality disorders, in a nationally representative sample of 12,312 US adults, aged 55 years and older, were collected from wave 2 of the National Epidemiologic Survey on Alcohol and Related Conditions.[9] The investigators found the youngest group, aged 55 to 64 years, had the highest prevalence (8.75%) of major depressive disorder (MDD) plus dysthymia. The prevalence of the depressive disorders declined as age increased (5.25% for ages 65–74 years, 4.41% for ages 75–84 years, and 5.0% for ages ≥85 years).[10] The investigators explained that the age difference of depression prevalence; that is, the leveling off in prevalence rates among adults aged 85 years and older, may be explained by the overall pattern of decreased prevalence of psychiatric disorders with increased age as in (1) the socioemotional selectivity theory[11] or (2) the strength and vulnerability integration theory.[12] The elderly who were reported having the lower prevalence of depression were generally without significant medical comorbidities. In reality, approximately 92% of older adults have at least 1 chronic disease and 77% have at least 2. Four chronic diseases (heart disease, cancer, stroke, and diabetes) cause almost two-thirds of all deaths each year. There are recognized causes leading to early-onset and late-onset depression (see **Table 1**). Clinically, however, many elderly depressed patients who had had remitted depression at younger ages and became depressed later in life. Care for these patients can be more challenging because these patients' biopsychosocial profiles tend to differ significantly from patients who have only late-onset depression. Therefore, knowing whether an elder person's depression may be a mixed type is important.

According the 2017 report from the Centers for Disease Control and Prevention, depression in older people living in the community ranges from less than 1% to about 5% but increases to 13.5% in those who require home health care and to 11.5% in older hospital patients.[13] Rates of depression may vary among different medical conditions. MDD and mild and subclinical depression have been found to be highly prevalent in patients with CVD. Abundant evidence suggests that approximately 15% to 20% of patients with ischemia heart disease and/or chronic heart failure experience MDD and another 15% to 20% of these patients may have subthreshold depressive symptoms.[14,15] Most cardiac subjects studied were older than 55 years.

Like a double-edged sword, comorbid depression and CVD hurt elder individuals bidirectionally in many aspects in their lives, with a synergetic impact. It is well known that individuals with depression have a higher incidence of CVD and individuals with CVD have a higher incidence of depression.[15,17] The impact of depression on the incidence of CVD events has been found to range from a relative risk of 2.3 to 5.4 in many studies. Greater prevalence of depression occurs in CVD patients and these patients experience greater mortality and medical morbidity compared with CVD patients without depression.[15,18] Depression also negatively affects quality of life, resulting in more social isolation, fragility, poor adherence to effective intervention and lifestyle modifications, the need for assistance with daily living, and so forth. Consequently, the health care expenditure for elderly individuals with CVD and depression grows into a major burden on the patients, their families, and society. For example, US expenditures on personal health care and public health in 2013 totaled $2.1 trillion, from which 14.39% was for CVD ($231.1 billion) and depressive disorders ($71.1 billion).[5] Older patients with depression have roughly 50% higher health care costs than nondepressed seniors.[5] Furthermore, depression is a significant predictor of suicide in elderly Americans. Comprising only 13% of the US population, individuals aged

65 years and older account for 20% of all suicide deaths, with white men being particularly vulnerable. Suicide among white men aged 85 years and older (65.3 deaths per 100,000 persons) is nearly 6 times the suicide rate (10.8 per 100,000) in the United States.[19]

DIAGNOSING DEPRESSION IN ELDERLY PATIENTS WITH CARDIOVASCULAR DISEASE

Depression is neither a normal response to life stress, nor a normal consequence of aging. It is a serious brain disease that can be effectively treated at any age if the treatment is appropriate. Symptomatology of depression can be easily assessed by the Patient Health Questionnaire, version 9, which can be easily self-administered by patients who are not cognitively compromised.[20] Unfortunately, symptoms of depression are often overlooked and untreated, especially when they coexist with other medical illnesses or life events that commonly occur as people age (eg, loss of loved ones). The following elements learned from the 1999 Mental Health America survey on attitudes and beliefs about clinical depression[19] may help in understanding this phenomenon:

- Approximately 68% of adults aged 65 years and older know little or almost nothing about depression.
- Only 38% of adults aged 65 years and older believe that depression is a health problem.
- If suffering from depression, older adults are more likely than any other group to handle it themselves. Only 42% would seek help from a health professional.
- Signs of depression are mentioned more frequently by people younger than age 64 years than by people aged 65 years and older. These include a change in eating habits (29% vs 15%), a change in sleeping habits (33% vs 16%), and sadness (28% vs 15%).
- About 58% of people aged 65 years and older believe that it is normal for people to get depressed as they grow older.

Several features must be kept in mind when making a diagnosis of depressive disorders in elderly individuals. Depression may present more subtly in the elderly, with patients frequently not endorsing low or depressed mood as the primary complaint, even if asked directly. Somatic complaints tend to overshadow the emotional struggles of elderly. Therefore, predominant somatic complaints, particularly when symptoms are diffuse, nonspecific, or chronic, that are not explained by revealing organic causes are often manifestations of underlying depression. Feeling overwhelmed, stressed out, and fatigued, and/or being burdened, is also highly suggestive of depression. Increased irritability, social withdrawal, or isolation may be signs of patients feeling they are unable to engage in tasks as they typically would, which is also a common sign of depression in the elderly. The early stages of depression are often not recognized in older patients; therefore, they may not be diagnosed until they reach more advanced stage; for example, when they have stopped eating, which may or may not be an expression of suicidal intent. Psychotic features, such as nihilistic and negativistic delusions, including themes of poverty and poor health, are common in older depressed patients. Prolonged or intensive grief from losses (of relationships, independence, health, comforts, activities; although grief can be a normal experience with advancing age), especially when accompanied by reduction of social interaction, food intake, and/or physical activities, deserves the attention of a mental care provider. Because active and passive suicidal ideation is common among elderly patients and difficult to detect, it is important for mental health professionals to be highly sensitive to signs of suicidal risk, especially for recently bereaved, isolated men who are in physical pain and drinking. Anxiety symptoms that may impede the appropriate diagnosis and management of depression tend to occur in elderly depressed patients.[21] Cognitive decline and dementia can mask the presentation of depression in the elderly who, at times, may have symptoms of pseudodementia as well. Obtaining collateral information from patients' family members or close friends is generally necessary when caring for depression in elderly patients.

Promptly diagnosing depression in patients with significant CVD can be more challenging because these patients rarely present to typical psychiatric care services and their physical symptoms are often hard to differentiate from depression. Financial constraints are also a significant factor preventing patients from receiving appropriate mental health care.

PATHOMECHANISMS UNDERLYING DEPRESSION AND CARDIOVASCULAR DISEASE IN THE ELDERLY

Several biological systems have been recognized to be dysfunctional and overlapping in CVD and in depression (**Fig. 1**). Aging is also associated with almost all of these identified dysfunctional features.[22] What may explain that approximately 50% of older adults have no CVD and depression? Investigations aimed at understanding the features and mechanisms of mental stress–induced myocardial ischemia or left ventricular dysfunction (MSILVD) have provided some helpful insight.

Mental stress tasks in a laboratory setting, such as a mental serial subtraction of 7 or giving a 3-minute speech about things that had been upsetting recently, trigger occurrence of MSILVD in approximately 50% of subjects who have clinically stable coronary heart disease (CHD).[22] Being a woman or living alone as a man increases the risk of having MSILVD. Alterations of C-reactive protein and cortisol in plasma induced by the mental stress tasks are associated with MSILVD. Also, mental stress task–induced

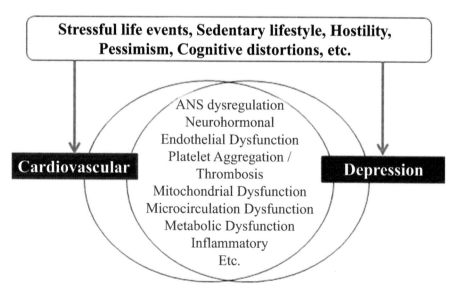

Fig. 1. Underlying pathomechanisms shared by depression and CVD in elderly. ANS, autonomic nerve system.

platelet hyperaggregation occurred in subjects with MSILVD.[23] Those clinically stable CHD subjects who responded normally to the challenge of mental tasks had no such alterations. Metabolomics research hinted that mental stress induced changes of metabolites reflecting mitochondrial dysregulation.[24] Resting measurements of these biomarkers, however, did not differ between subjects who had normal responses and patients who developed MSILVD to mental tasks (unpublished data). Multiple investigations demonstrate symptoms of depression are associated with development of MSILVD.[22] MSILVD has been found consistently to be a significant and independent predictor for adverse CVD outcomes in clinically stable CHD patients.[25]

MSILVD investigations have revealed a critical interwoven mechanism underlying the adversity of CVD with comorbid depression. Such investigations, in addition, are reminders that certain patients' cardiovascular systems will respond to commonly encountered mental stressors more adversely than others. Mental stress–induced dynamic changes indicate that application of mental stress testing may be an effective measure to identify individuals who are more susceptible to emotional stressful experiences.

IMPROVING THE CARE FOR ELDERLY PATIENTS WITH CARDIOVASCULAR DISEASE AND DEPRESSION

Depression in the elderly seems to respond to common pharmacologic and psychosocial-behavioral interventions as effectively as that in younger individuals.[27] Bartels and colleagues[26] provide a thorough overview of empirically validated treatments and conclude that antidepressants are generally effective for treating geriatric depression, with most studies showing that more than half of older adults treated with antidepressants experience at least a 50% reduction in depressive symptoms. Furthermore, these investigators report that cognitive-behavioral therapy has the greatest empirical support for effectiveness in the treatment of geriatric depression among several forms of psychosocial interventions, such as problem-solving therapy, interpersonal therapy, brief psychodynamic therapy, and reminiscence therapy. Moreover, evidence suggests that a combination of pharmacologic and psychosocial interventions is more effective than either intervention alone in preventing recurrence of MDD,[27] especially when a clearly identified psychosocial stressor is at the root of its cause.

Promptly identifying depression and beginning appropriate interventions are essential components for the care of elderly CVD patients. There are usually 3 phases for the intervention to successfully achieve the effective care for these patients:

1. An acute treatment phase to achieve remission of depression
2. A continuation phase to prevent recurrence of depression (relapse)
3. A maintenance (prophylaxis) phase to prevent future episodes (recurrence).[28]

In addition, the following elements must be considered.

First, the key principle is to appropriately select antidepressants with the goal of ascertaining the safety of these patients who tend to be on polypharmacy and experience alterations in normal drug metabolism and elimination. Selective serotonin reuptake inhibitors (SSRIs) are recommended as the first-line choice of antidepressants because they are generally considered safe for CVD patients. However, there are 4 critical points to consider when choosing a particular antidepressant. Patients who have or are susceptible for prolongation of corrected QT interval must avoid citalopram and escitalopram.[16] Adverse drug-drug interaction can be common in elderly patients and usually requires a thorough review of medications, including health supplements and close monitoring of unanticipated symptoms. The Flockhart Table, or P450 Drug Interaction Table, consists of detailed cytochrome P (CYP) 450 enzyme-related drug interactions (available at http://medicine.iupui.edu/clinpharm/ddis/clinical-table). Fluoxetine has a long half-life and, therefore, should be avoided if frequent medication change is an issue for a patient. Although most adverse effects caused by SSRIs are short-lasting, the sexual dysfunction of SSRIs needs to be clearly discussed with these elderly patients without assuming that they do not care about their sexuality. Initiating a lower dose of the recommended drug for nonmedically ill patients tends to minimize adverse effects. Other antidepressants, such as venlafaxine, duloxetine, bupropion, and mirtazapine, may be considered as single agents, or as augmentation for the treatment of depression in CVD patients. However, close monitoring of blood pressure and heart rate with those medications may be required, especially when the doses are altered. Tricyclic antidepressants should be avoided owing to the known cardiac conduction system[16] adverse effects of these medications.

Second, depression in elderly CVD patients tends to be chronic with fluctuation from milder to severe. Therefore, preparing patients and their loved ones for committing to long-term intervention and aiming at functional improvement rather than simple symptom reduction may enhance the compliance and effectiveness of the intervention.

Third, despite the previously mentioned interventions, patients' depression may regress. Therefore, the clinician must be sensitive to certain symptoms, such as notable reduction of interaction with family, eating little or nothing, reduced verbal communication (even muteness), or being delusional, which may warrant medical and/or mental hospitalization and/or receiving electroconvulsive interventions.

There is evidence indicating that SSRIs may have cardiovascular protective effects, though several clinical trials have not been able to show that SSRIs improve CVD outcomes.[29] It was demonstrated that 6 weeks of escitalopram resulted in about 2.5 times reduction of MSILVD compared with the matched placebo in clinically stable CHD subjects.[29] Kamarck and colleagues[30] reported 2-month citalopram favorably changed metabolic risk factors, such as waist circumference ($P = .003$), glucose ($P = .02$), high-density lipoprotein cholesterol ($P = .04$), triglycerides ($P = .03$), insulin sensitivity ($P = .045$), and diastolic blood pressure by automated assessment ($P = .0021$) compared with placebo in 159 healthy adults with elevated hostility scores.

Regardless of the pharmacologic therapy chosen, it is important to consider the psychological, social, and environmental context of each patient. Various psychosocial behavioral interventions, such as life review, exercise,[31] music therapy, stress management,[31] and many others,[18] benefit the elderly. Tailoring interventions to the needs and acceptance of particular individuals can be challenging but necessary, especially in consideration of the accessibility and resources of each patient. Establishing tangible plans with the patients and their loved ones can be invaluable.

Integrated collaborative care with a systematic approach and targeting effective primary and secondary preventions has been considered most cost-effective in caring for medically ill patients with comorbid depression and other mental health conditions[32] but implementation of such caring mechanisms may take time to be effective.

In summary, comorbid CVD and depression constitutes a huge challenge for these patients, their loved ones, health providers, and the entire society globally. Greater attention, effort, and resources with integrated collaboration are needed to overcome this upcoming disastrous matter.

REFERENCES

1. Wan He, Daniel Goodkind, and Paul Kowal (2016). An Aging World: 2015 International Population Reports (Issued March 2016 P95/16–1). Available at:

https://www.census.gov/content/dam/Census/library/publications/2016/demo/p95-16-1.pdf. Accessed November 24, 2017.

2. Fact sheet: aging in the United States (2016). Available at: http://www.prb.org/Publications/Media-Guides/2016/aging-unitedstates-fact-sheet.aspx. Accessed June 10, 2017.

3. Prince MJ, Wu F, Guo Y, et al. The burden of disease in older people and implications for health policy and practice. Lancet 2015;385(9967):549–62.

4. Mozaffarian D, Benjamin EJ, Go AS, et al, on behalf of the American Heart Association Statistics Committee and Stroke Statistics Subcommittee. Heart disease and stroke statistics—2016 update: a report from the American Heart Association. Circulation 2016;133:e38–360.

5. Dieleman JL, Baral R, Birger M, et al. US spending on personal health care and public health, 1996-2013. JAMA 2016;316(24):2627–46.

6. American Association of Geriatric Psychiatry (2008). Geriatrics and mental health—the facts. Available at: http://www.aagponline.org/prof/facts_mh.asp. Accessed June 23, 2008.

7. Bukh JD, Bock C, Vinberg M, et al. Differences between early and late onset adult depression. Clin Pract Epidemiol Ment Health 2011;7:140–7.

8. Blazer DG. Depression in late life: review and commentary. J Gerontol A Biol Sci Med Sci 2003;58:249–65.

9. Hasin DS, Grant BF. The national epidemiologic survey on alcohol and related conditions (NESARC) waves 1 and 2: review and summary of findings. Soc Psychiatry Psychiatr Epidemiol 2015;50:1609–40.

10. Reynolds K, Pietrzak RH, El-Gabalawy R, et al. Prevalence of psychiatric disorders in U.S. older adults: findings from a nationally representative survey. World Psychiatry 2015;14:74–81.

11. Carstensen LL, Isaacowitz DM, Charles ST. Taking time seriously: a theory of socioemotional electivity. Am Psychol 1999;54:165–81.

12. Charles ST. Strength and vulnerability integration: a model of emotional well-being across adulthood. Psychol Bull 2010;136:1068–91.

13. CDC 2017. Available at: https://www.cdc.gov/aging/mentalhealth/depression.htm. Accessed May 15, 2017.

14. Jiang W, Alexander J, Christopher E, et al. Relationship of depression to increased risk of mortality and rehospitalization in patients with congestive heart failure. Arch Intern Med 2001;161:1849–56.

15. Jiang W, Krishnan RR, O'Connor CM. Depression and heart disease: evidence of a link, and its therapeutic implications. CNS Drugs 2002;16:111–27.

16. Khawaja IS, Westermeyer JJ, Gajwani P, et al. Depression and coronary artery disease: the association, mechanisms, and therapeutic implications. Psychiatry (Edgmont) 2009;6:38–51.

17. Rozanski A. Behavioral cardiology: current advances and future directions. J Am Coll Cardiol 2014;64:100–10.

18. National Institute of Mental Health: older adults: depression and suicide fact sheet. Accessed August 1999. Netscape: Available at: http://www.nimh.nih.gov/publicat/elderlydepsuicide.cfm. Accessed on June 10, 2017.

19. Haddad M, Walters P, Phillips R, et al. Detecting depression in patients with coronary heart disease: a diagnostic evaluation of the PHQ-9 and HADS-D in primary care, findings from the UPBEAT-UK study. PLoS One 2013;8(10):e78493.

20. King-Kallimanis B, Gum A, Kohn R. Comorbidity of depressive and anxiety disorders for older Americans in the national comorbidity survey-replication. Am J Geriatr Psychiatry 2009;17:782–92.

21. Paneni F, Diaz Cañestro C, Libby P, et al. The aging cardiovascular system: understanding it at the cellular and clinical levels. J Am Coll Cardiol 2017;69: 1952–67.
22. Jiang W. Emotional triggering of cardiac dysfunction: the present and future. Curr Cardiol Rep 2015;17:635.
23. Jiang W, Samad Z, Boyle S, et al. Prevalence and clinical characteristics of mental stress-induced myocardial ischemia in patients with coronary heart disease. J Am Coll Cardiol 2013;61:714–22.
24. Boyle SH, Matson WR, Eric J, on behalf of the REMIT Investigators. Metabolomics analysis reveals insights into biochemical mechanisms of mental stress-induced left ventricular dysfunction. Metabolomics 2015;11(3):571–82.
25. Sun JL, Boyle SH, Samad Z, et al. Mental stress-induced left ventricular dysfunction and adverse outcome in ischemic heart disease patients. Eur J Prev Cardiol 2017;24:591–9.
26. Bartels SJ, Dums AR, Oxman TE, et al. Evidence-based practices in geriatric mental health care: an overview of systematic reviews and meta-analyses. Psychiatr Clin North Am 2003;26(4):971–90, x–xi.
27. Alexopoulos GS, Katz IR, Bruce ML, et al. Remission in depressed geriatric primary care patients: a report from the PROSPECT study. Am J Psychiatry 2005; 162(4):718–24.
28. Echols MR, Jiang W. Clinical trial evidence for treatment of depression in heart failure. Heart Fail Clin 2011;7:81–8.
29. Jiang W, Velazquez EJ, Kuchibhatla M, et al. Responses of mental stress-induced myocardial ischemia to escitalopram treatment: results from the REMIT trial. JAMA 2013;309:2139–49.
30. Kamarck TW, Muldoon MF, Manuck SB, et al. Citalopram improves metabolic risk factors among high hostile adults: results of a placebo-controlled intervention. Psychoneuroendocrinology 2011;36:1070–9.
31. Blumenthal JA, Sherwood A, Babyak MA, et al. Effects of exercise and stress management training on markers of cardiovascular risk in patients with ischemic heart disease: a randomized controlled trial. JAMA 2005;293(13):1626–34.
32. Katon WJ, Lin EH, Von Korff M, et al. Collaborative care for patients with depression and chronic illnesses. N Engl J Med 2010;363:2611–20.

Advances in the Conceptualization and Study of Schizophrenia in Later Life

 CrossMark

Carl I. Cohen, MD*, Ksenia Freeman, MD, Dina Ghoneim, MD,
Aninditha Vengassery, MD, Brian Ghezelaiagh, BA,
Michael M. Reinhardt, MD

KEYWORDS

- Schizophrenia and older adults • Remission in schizophrenia in later life
- Paradoxical aging and schizophrenia • Accelerated aging and schizophrenia

KEY POINTS

- Point prevalence data indicate that approximately half of older adults with schizophrenia (OAS) are in clinical remission and one-quarter achieve community integration concomitantly with clinical remission.
- Longitudinally, persistent remission is less common (one-fourth) and the persistence of both remission and community integration is infrequent (one-eighth).
- For many persons, recovery continues into later life and is an ongoing process in which some persons improve with respect to remission and/or social integration and some worsen over time.
- There are clinical and physiologic reasons to suggest that doses of antipsychotic medications can be reduced or, in some instances, eliminated.

INTRODUCTION

The aim of this article is to provide an overview of the advances in the conceptualization and study of schizophrenia in later life. In so doing, theoretical and clinical models in psychiatry and gerontology are integrated. Specifically, recovery is examined in the context of aging, how clinical dimensionality affects diagnoses in older adults, how various features of schizophrenia are implicated in models of accelerated and paradoxical aging, and how outcome in later life is a more dynamic and heterogeneous than assumed previously.

Disclosure: The authors have nothing to disclose.
Department of Psychiatry, SUNY Downstate Medical Center, Brooklyn, NY, USA
* Corresponding author. Division of Geriatric Psychiatry, SUNY Downstate Medical Center, MSC1203, 450 Clarkson Avenue, Brooklyn, NY 11203-2098.
E-mail address: carl.cohen@downstate.edu

Psychiatr Clin N Am 41 (2018) 39–53
https://doi.org/10.1016/j.psc.2017.10.004
0193-953X/18/© 2017 Elsevier Inc. All rights reserved.

BACKGROUND: DEFINITIONS AND EPIDEMIOLOGY
Age Criteria

There is no consensus on what age demarcates older adults with schizophrenia (OAS), and this has made comparisons between studies difficult. Because of the appreciably shortened life span of persons with schizophrenia,[1] many researchers have used younger ages for study. Thus, age cutoffs of 50, 55, and 60 are common, and in some instances investigators have used samples that combined middle-age (ages 40 and over) with older participants.

Age of Onset

Approximately 20% to 25% of patients with schizophrenia have an onset of the disorder after age 40.[2] A Dutch case register study of persons ages 60 and over found 64% had early-onset schizophrenia,[3] suggesting that the loss of early-onset individuals (to death or recovery) may be compensated for by the influx of cases with a later onset. There has been considerable historical vacillation in diagnostic criteria regarding age of onset.[4] The early editions of the *Diagnostic and Statistical Manual of Mental Disorders (DSM)* did not specify age of onset criteria for schizophrenia. The first edition of the *DSM* and the *DSM* (Second Edition) included the category "Involutional Psychotic Reaction" for psychotic symptoms occurring during the involutional period, and the *DSM* (Second Edition) used the terms, "involutional state" and "involutional paraphrenia," to describe a delusional condition with onset during the involutional period. In contradistinction, the *DSM* (Third Edition) (*DSM-III*) restricted the diagnosis of schizophrenia to onset before age 45, whereas the *DSM-III* (Revised) included a late-onset category for initial presentations after age 44. The *International Statistical Classification of Diseases (ICD), Ninth Revision*, included a diagnosis of "Paraphrenia" and listed "Involutional Paranoid State" and "Paraphrenia, Involutional" as approximate synonyms. The *ICD, Tenth Revision*; *DSM* (Fourth Edition); *DSM* (Fourth Edition, Text Revision); and *DSM* (Fifth Edition) (*DSM-5*) did not include separate diagnostic categories or criteria for late-onset schizophrenia.

The omission of a late-life category is problematic because there is evidence that late-onset disorders, especially those arising after age 60, may differ from earlier-onset cases. In 2000, an international expert group published a consensus report that proposed that schizophrenia be termed, "Late-Onset Schizophrenia" and "Very-Late-Onset Schizophrenia-Like Psychosis," for disorders that have an onset between ages 40 and 60 and after age 60, respectively.[5] When the disorder arises between ages 40 and 60, it has been thought to resemble the early-onset subtype, although there are modest differences, such as a preponderance of women, a lower level of symptom severity, and less executive dysfunction.[6] The very-late-onset subtype is distinguished by many more women; higher rates of visual, tactile, and olfactory hallucinations; greater prevalence of persecutory and partition delusions; absence of formal thought disorder or negative symptoms; lower genetic load; and possibly higher standard mortality rate versus older persons with early-onset disorder, primarily due to higher rates of comorbid illness and accidents.[5,7] Comparisons between studies have been made more difficult because these age categories often have been conflated.

Epidemiology

Estimates from the United States and the United Kingdom place the prevalence for schizophrenia at 0.6% to 1% in persons ages 45 and over and 0.1% to 0.5% in persons ages 65 and over.[8] In the United States, by 2025, 1.1 million people or approximately one-fourth of all persons with schizophrenia will be ages 55 and over.[9] Globally, the number of persons 60 and over will double by 2050, with estimates reaching more than 10 million persons with schizophrenia.[10] A crisis looms as research and clinical programs have not kept pace with these demographic shifts. A PubMed search indicates that less than 1% of the literature on schizophrenia has been devoted to older adults.

Cohen and coauthors[10] observed that there are now 2 generations of older OAS, who may require different therapeutic interventions: (1) the old-old (those ages 75 and over), who typically experienced many years of institutionalization before entering the community and face substantial cognitive and physical problems, and (2) the young-old (ages 55–74), who have had briefer hospitalizations and been exposed to recovery service models that have been more focused on consumer needs and personal autonomy. The young-old also have higher rates of physical and cognitive deficits than age-matched controls, albeit less severe than the older counterparts.[10] In the United States, more than 85% of older persons with schizophrenia are living in a range of settings in the community whereas the remainder live in long-term hospitals or nursing homes.[9] The population found in long-term care settings has the most severe outcomes and more closely resembles those individuals described by Kraepelin as having "dementia praecox."[11]

RECOVERY MODEL AND OLDER ADULTS WITH SCHIZOPHRENIA

The Substance Abuse and Mental Health Services Administration conceptualizes recovery as "A process of change through which individuals improve their health and wellness, live a self-directed life, and strive to reach their full potential."[12] Recovery in OAS can be conceptualized as a pathway moving from clinical remission and community integration (together termed "objective recovery") to a positive state of aging (successful aging). Until recently, the course of schizophrenia in later life was largely viewed as a quiescent or stable end stage.[2] As described later, however, it is now recognized that there is considerable fluctuation in various clinical and psychosocial indicators. Thus, in many instances, there are opportunities for further recovery in later life.[2] Conversely, there is also the potential for decline. In either case, it is important to appreciate the value of clinical and psychosocial interventions to prevent regression and foster improvement. In this section, the prospects for recovery at different stages in the model are described.

Symptomatic Remission

For most of the twentieth century, schizophrenia was thought to have an ominous prognosis, with fewer than one-fifth of persons likely to show any clinical improvement. Kraepelin postulated a recovery rate of 2.6% to 4.1% and a 17% improvement rate.[13] The *DSM-III*[14] stated, "The most common course is one of acute exacerbations with increasing impairment between episodes." In the late 1970s and 1980s, however, the publication of studies of hospitalized persons who were assessed after several decades resulted in a revision in prognosis: half to two-thirds of persons were found to have significant clinical improvement in later life.[10] More recently, based on an adaptation of the remission criteria by the Remission in Schizophrenia Working Group,[15] 3 cross-sectional studies of community-dwelling OAS found remission rates of approximately 50% in early-onset schizophrenia patients in the United States, whereas a catchment-area based study in the Netherlands (including some institutionalized patients and late-onset cases) reported a 29% symptom remission rate.[16–18] The International Study of Schizophrenia comprising 18 worldwide cohorts found that on 15-year or 25-year follow-up, 54% of those in the prevalence group (mean age

51 years) were symptom-free or had nondisabling residual symptoms.[19] Persons in developing countries generally had better outcomes than in developed ones.

Recently, a longitudinal study (mean 52 months) in New York City by Cohen and Iqbal,[20] comprising 104 older adults ages 55 and over with early-onset schizophrenia spectrum disorder, found that although there was a nonsignificant decline in the point prevalence attaining symptom remission (49% baseline; 40% follow-up), only 25% were in remission at both assessments; 35% were not in remission at either assessment; 25% went from remission to nonremission; and 16% went from nonremission to remission. These findings suggest a recalibration with respect to late-life outcome from one of excessive optimism based on cross-sectional data (50% symptom clinical remission) to a more nuanced view of involving the potential for movement in either clinical direction, with two-fifths of persons shifting clinical remission statuses.

Community Integration

Community integration is a comprehensive social indicator that is an important component of the gerontological recovery model, occurring in tandem with clinical remission and preceding successful aging.[21] It can be viewed as normalization of functioning in society and comprises assessments of functioning and perceived quality of life (QOL) within several dimensions, namely, independence, physical health, psychological well-being, and social integration. In a cross-sectional study in New York City, OAS scored lower than a community comparison group on each of the 4 dimensions of the 12-item community integration scale.[22] Community-living older adults had approximately twice the level of high community integration (positive scores of 10 or more items) than the schizophrenia group (41% vs 23%). In a longitudinal study, the persons with schizophrenia using the same sample,[23] 39% remained in the low community integration group at both points in time, 26% were in the high community integration group at both assessments, and 36% of persons fluctuated between high and low community integration. Thus, although most older people with schizophrenia have diminished social functioning versus their healthy age peers, there is considerable heterogeneity, ranging from severely incapacitated functioning and socially isolated individuals to near-normal functioning and socially integrated persons[24]; there are opportunities for improvement but also risks for decline.

Our group's analysis of data derived from the New York City sample described previously,[16,20,22,23] indicated that 26% of persons attained concurrent clinical remission and high community integration at baseline; ie, "objective recovery". Only 12% of the sample simultaneously attained clinical remission and high community integration at both points in time; on the other hand, only 18% experienced no clinical remission and had low community integration at both assessments. Thus, 7 in 10 persons had some combination of the remission and community integration, sometimes reflecting changes in these parameters over time.

Successful Aging

Geriatric medicine and psychiatry have increasingly broadened their perspectives from disability and disease to positive health and well-being. In later life, the latter is sometimes termed, *successful aging*, and is viewed as a state involving the absence of disability accompanied by high physical, cognitive, and social functioning.[25] Successful aging is an ideal that all older persons might achieve under optimal circumstances. In looking at the percentage of OAS who achieved successful aging, Ibrahim and colleagues[25] found that only 2% met all 6 criteria whereas 19% of community comparison group attained this level, which was similar to the mean rate found in other geriatric studies.[26] Thus, successful aging, which is found in only a minority of normal community elders, is an unlikely outcome among OAS.

DEPRESSION IN OLDER ADULTS WITH SCHIZOPHRENIA

Among middle-aged and older persons with schizophrenia living in the community, the cross-sectional prevalence rates of depression have ranged from 44% to 75%.[27–32] These studies found associations between depressive symptoms and psychotic symptoms, decreased level of functioning, increased overall psychopathology, severity of general medical conditions, decreased QOL, diminished social contacts, and diminished use of several healthy coping strategies, often at levels below the criteria for major depression. A related concern is suicidality in older OAS. Although rates of suicide diminish in later life, they still remain higher than their age peers.[33] Cohen and colleagues[34] found a significantly higher prevalence of current suicidality among OAS compared with a comparison group (10% vs 2%) as well as past suicidal attempts (30% vs 4%); 19% of those who previously attempted suicide still exhibited suicidality. Among those who expressed suicidality, 70% were clinically depressed, although not necessarily meeting criteria for major depression, versus 28% of those without suicidality.

A prospective study[35] of OAS from the New York City sample found fluidity in symptoms in many persons: 26% fluctuated between depression and nondepression; persistent depression (defined as either syndromal or subsyndromal depression) occurred in 44% of persons; and 30% remained persistently nondepressed. These findings challenged the notion that schizophrenia in later life is typically characterized by affective withdrawal or quiescence.[36,37]

These fluctuations of mood have raised questions regarding the feasibility and clinical relevance of diagnosing schizoaffective disorder in OAS (which requires a diagnosis of major mood disorder for a majority of the total duration of active and residual portion of the illness).[38] Most studies of OAS have combined persons with schizophrenia and schizoaffective disorder under the broader category of "schizophrenia spectrum disorders." Although *DSM-5* did not incorporate the dimensional approach into the body of the manual, it seems especially germane to OAS because aging persons often display symptoms of depression that do not meet the criteria of a major clinical disorder but nevertheless have important implications for health and daily functioning.

ACCELERATED AGING

Accelerated aging refers to an increased physical morbidity and mortality along with possible declines in cognition and augmented levels of aging biomarkers found in persons with schizophrenia.[39,40] Accelerated aging in schizophrenia can be examined from various perspectives, such as cognition, physical disease, mortality rates, brain structure, and various biomarkers.

Cognition

Within the accelerated aging model, cognitive decline is a controversial area. It is well established that OAS have more cognitive deficits than their age-matched peers. In a recent study of schizophrenia, persons ages 50 and over had cognitive deficits nearly 2 SDs below control participants.[41] Rajji and coauthors[42] found that compared with healthy controls, persons with schizophrenia, ages 19 to 79, had lower overall cognition scores as well as in all other cognitive domains except for social cognition. The rate of decline across the age groups was similar to that observed in the healthy control groups. Consequently, schizophrenia is no longer viewed as a neurodegenerative disorder (dementia praecox) but rather a neurodevelopmental disorder in which deficits arise around the time of onset and do not progress beyond the expected effect of aging. Although the rate of cognitive decline in schizophrenia may be similar to that in age-matched controls, the preexisting deficits accrued at disease onset result in an earlier crossing of the threshold into major neurocognitive impairment (dementia).

Longitudinal data suggest heterogeneous cognitive trajectories. Within-group longitudinal data of middle-aged and older OAS in the community showed considerable heterogeneity: a majority of persons seemed cognitively stable; however, approximately one-fifth showed more rapid decline and one-fifth showed improvement, often rising from dementia to near-normal levels.[43,44] Worse cognition (global and/or domain-specific) has been found strongly associated with diminished functional competence and community adaptation as well as with greater age, female gender, lower education, living in an institution, longer duration of illness, earlier age of onset, and higher levels of positive and negative symptoms.[5,45]

Using data of older persons (mean age 70) derived from an urban public health system, Hendrie and coauthors[46] found significantly higher rates of dementia in persons with schizophrenia (64%) versus those without schizophrenia (32%), although the investigators conjectured that some persons may have been misdiagnosed. A Danish registry[47] study also found 2-times greater risk of dementia in persons with schizophrenia, although the prevalence rates at age 65 were low (1.8% for schizophrenia vs 0.6% for nonschizophrenia groups). Of 3 community-based longitudinal studies, 2 reported an increased prevalence of dementia and 1 did not.[48] Friedman and coinvestigators[49] found accelerated cognitive decline experienced by chronically institutionalized persons with schizophrenia beginning at age 65, but the decline in cognition was substantially less than in Alzheimer disease (AD). Patterns of decline, neuropathology, and polygenetic findings, even among more chronically hospitalized groups, did not resemble those of AD. Moreover, Rajji and associates'[50] review of older schizophrenia patients concluded that the findings of cognitive decline at age 65 found in institutionalized persons do not seem to apply to those who have been living in the community.

Finally, many OAS, because they have early cognitive impairment, and show a gradual lifetime decline in cognition that results in their classification as having a major neurocognitive disorder in later life. Is this really a new clinical disorder or is it a dimensional component of the schizophrenia? The facts that the course of decline and the underlying neuropathology differ from AD and that one-fifth of persons show substantial improvements in cognition over time suggest that in most instances rendering a diagnosis of major neurocognitive disorder may be inappropriate. As in the case of depression, the use of the dimensional perspective described in the *DSM-5* appendix can be helpful in resolving these diagnostic issues.

Physical Illness and Mortality Rates

Life expectancy is reduced 15 years to 20 years for people with schizophrenia.[1] The mortality risk in schizophrenia is 2-times to 3-times higher than in the general population, and this differential mortality gap has increased in recent decades.[51] Although persons with early-onset schizophrenia who live into old age should be considered survivors, the differential in mortality rates between persons with schizophrenia and their age peers persists into later life, perhaps even into their 80s.[46,52,53] Although the mortality rate from suicides and accidents is elevated in older individuals with schizophrenia, natural causes of death account for the largest part of the reduction in life expectancy.[52,54] Greater mortality rates are thought to reflect the high prevalence of cardiovascular disease, diabetes, and metabolic syndrome that partially can be attributed to lifestyle factors (smoking, poor dietary habits, and limited physical activity) and the effects of antipsychotic medications, especially those in the second-generation group. Part of the excess morbidity and mortality, however, may be inherent to the disorder itself and there has been interest in searching for evidence of inflammation and oxidative stress.[40]

In contrast to schizophrenia at a younger age, few studies have looked into the physical comorbidities of OAS. Hendrie and colleagues[46] found that compared with their age peers, OAS had significantly higher rates of congestive heart failure, chronic obstructive pulmonary disease, and hypothyroidism, whereas they had lower cancer rates. Kredentser and coauthors[54] found deaths from cancer higher among middle-aged persons with schizophrenia but not in persons over age 59.

OAS may be at risk for undetected or inadequately treated medical conditions that may be a consequence of systemic or individual factors.[55] A recent Danish registry study[56] found that OAS ages 70 and over did not differ from controls with regard to registered chronic medical illnesses but were significantly less likely to receive medication for cardiovascular diseases; hospital admissions and number of days hospitalized were equal to controls but with significantly fewer general medical outpatient contacts. Findings of older persons with schizophrenia have mirrored those in younger samples, indicating that schizophrenia itself may pose a barrier to accessing adequate health care due to worse compliance or diminished understanding of symptoms and illness management.[55,57]

Biomarkers of Aging

Nguyen and colleagues'[58] review found that a majority of studies reported abnormal biomarker levels among individuals with schizophrenia, including senescence-related indices of inflammation, telomere length, oxidative stress, metabolic health, gene expression, synaptic function, and testosterone, suggesting that schizophrenia is associated with aging-related biochemical abnormalities; 26% of the studies observed differential age-related decline in schizophrenia. Markers of receptor/synaptic function and gene expression were most frequently differentially related to age. Schizophrenia patients with greater disease severity and longer illness duration exhibited higher levels of inflammatory and oxidative stress biomarkers and shorter telomere length. These studies have been limited by cross-sectional design, small sample sizes, and failure to control for potentially confounding variables, especially factors such as smoking, substance abuse, exercise, diet, and access to health care.

Brain Structure

Numerous cross-sectional studies support structural brain alterations in schizophrenia patients and controls: gray matter reductions in frontal, temporal, and postcentral cortical regions, and increased ventricular size and white matter reductions in the corpus callosum, although these findings have been inconsistent and sometimes of poor quality.[59] Heilbronner and coauthors'[60] review of longitudinal neuroimaging studies concluded that whole-brain volume does not differ over time; however, there may be progressive decreases in gray matter and possibly in white matter; functional MRI changes are affected by symptomatology. The investigators caution that longitudinal studies in the field of neuroimaging typically have durations limited to only a few years and rarely beyond 6 years. Thus, their relevance to older adults is unknown. A recent longitudinal study by Schnack and colleagues[61] comparing MRI scans for healthy subjects and persons with schizophrenia (age range 16–67 years) found that there was an "accelerated" pattern of brain aging in schizophrenia persons at illness onset and during the initial 5 years; after that time period, the rates of decline were comparable between the 2 groups, although the brain gap stayed constant. Hahn and colleagues'[62] review of neuroimaging studies that compared early-onset and late-onset schizophrenia reported differences in 8 of 10 studies, but these were not consistent across studies.

PARADOXIC AGING

Paradoxic aging refers to the concurrent decline in physical health and some cognitive functions with an improvement in subjective QOL and psychosocial functioning.[39] This paradox is believed even more pronounced in OAS, in which there are higher rates of mortality and physical disease in tandem with a trend toward fewer relapses, increased rates of clinical remission, and better self-management. Many older OAS successfully adapt to the illness, with increased use of positive coping techniques, enhanced self-esteem, and increased social support.

Quality of Life

Jeste and coauthors[39] astutely observed, "For most people with schizophrenia, QOL is a more meaningful outcome than psychiatric symptoms and cognition." In younger and broad age range studies of persons with schizophrenia, there is evidence that QOL can serve as a predictor of symptomatic and functional improvement. Thus, identifying factors that can affect QOL has important implications for clinical practice. Depression and cognitive impairment have been the variables most commonly associated with lower QOL in cross-sectional studies of OAS.[63,64] Like other clinical and social variables, QOL is not always stable over time. In the New York City sample described previously, 28% moved between high and low categories on follow-up, whereas 32% and 40% of the sample were in the high and low QOL categories, respectively, at both points in time.[64]

Social Functioning

A review by Meesters and colleagues[24] concluded, "The majority of older schizophrenic patients are well behind their healthy age peers with respect to various aspects of social functioning such as social roles, social support, and social skills." At the same time considerable heterogeneity among patients can be found, and cognitive functioning had a major impact on social functioning, outweighing clinical symptoms.

Coping Strategies

A variety of researchers have expressed optimism on the potential for healing in aging persons with schizophrenia. Bleuler[65] proffered the following dictum: "The healthy life of schizophrenics is never extinguished." In a qualitative study of middle-aged and older OAS, Shepherd and colleagues[66] found that early in the course of their illness participants experienced confusion about diagnosis, active psychotic symptoms, and withdrawal/losses in social networks. Thereafter, nearly all believed that their symptoms had improved, which they attributed to increased skills in self-management of positive symptoms. There was marked heterogeneity in perceptions about functioning, however. Some participants were in despair about the discrepancy between their current situations and life goals (31%), many were resigned to remain in supported environments (50%), and others were working toward functional attainments and were optimistic about the future (19%).[66]

Martinsson and colleagues[67] found the focus of OAS narratives was on "struggling for existence," which was characterized as a loss of dignity of identity, feeling troubled and powerless, and yearning for respect. The older persons fought to master their existence and to be seen for who they are. Likewise, Avieli and colleagues[68] identified 9 dimensions of suffering: social rejection, familial rejection, the symptoms of schizophrenia, hospitalization, the side effects of medication, loss of employment potential, loss of independent accommodation, loss of social life, and loss of hope about becoming a partner and a parent. Additionally, the suffering of OAS seemed cumulative and often accompanied by ongoing feelings of loneliness and stigma. The nature of the life story work at this stage of their lives was characterized by the struggle between achieving normative life goals and suffering the consequences of schizophrenia.

With respect to developing coping strategies, Cohen and coauthors[69] found coping styles used by OAS to deal with life stressors were similar to their age peers. Both groups most commonly used cognitive coping strategies (eg, accept situation and keep sense of humor), and at equivalent levels. With respect to troubling symptoms, OAS often redirected their attention by using a wide range of coping strategies. Behavioral strategies were the most frequently used methods to manage symptoms; also, "acceptance" of and "fighting back" against symptoms showed positive and negative trends, respectively, with increased age.[70,71] Finally, psychotic symptoms may have a salutary effect on resiliency and coping with daily hassles. Cohen and colleagues[72] found that the percentage of persons hearing pleasant or good voices and obeying voices was higher in OAS than in younger samples. If older persons heard good voices, they were 3.5-times more likely to obey orders than if they heard bad voices, suggesting a potentially healthy coping strategy to deal with the persistence of voices in later life.

TREATMENT

There is surprisingly little written about first-line treatment and recommended dosages in OAS with early-onset. With respect to the late-onset disorder, a Cochrane report,[73] updated in 2012, concluded that there is a paucity of trial-based evidence on which to base guidelines for the treatment of late-onset schizophrenia and that there is a need for good quality-controlled clinical trials. Khan and colleagues[74] provided an update on an earlier consensus article by Alexopoulus and coauthors.[75] The original report recommended risperidone (1.25–3.5 mg/d) as first-line treatment of late-life schizophrenia; the second-line treatments are quetiapine (100–300 mg/d), olanzapine (7.5–15 mg/d), and aripiprazole (15–30 mg/d). The starting dose for antipsychotics should be one-quarter of the typical adult dose and the maintenance dose is typically one-third to one-half of the adult dose.

There have been 2 double-blind studies using raloxifene in postmenopausal women with schizophrenia. One study found a greater reduction in general and total Positive and Negative Syndrome Scale (PANSS) score over placebo (but not in the positive or negative symptom subscale scores) and an increased probability of clinical response over placebo[76]; the second study found reduced general, total, and negative PANSS scores but not positive subscale scores.[77] One controlled study suggested that citalopram may be effective for treating middle-aged and older schizophrenia adults with subsyndromal depression.[78]

A literature review of electroconvulsive therapy (ECT) in OAS identified 6 prospective studies and 1 case series; participants were between 49 years and 96 years old.[79] The investigators concluded that bilateral ECT seemed effective as an acute and maintenance treatment of OAS who had the onset of their illness earlier in life. ECT was not effective in those with very-late-onset psychosis possibly due to the high prevalence of comorbid brain pathology other than schizophrenia. Transcranial magnetic stimulation and deep brain stimulation have not been studied in OAS.

There have been numerous concerns regarding the long-term use of medications. OAS show vulnerability to adverse effects of medications (eg, cardiovascular, metabolic, anticholinergic, and extrapyramidal effects; orthostasis; sedation; falls; and neuroleptic malignant syndrome) that result from pharmacokinetic and pharmacodynamic changes associated with aging. Moreover, in a middle-aged sample (mean age: 43 years), higher lifetime antipsychotic dose-years were associated with poorer cognitive performance.[80] Similarly, Rajii and coauthors[81] found that reducing the antipsychotic dose resulted in increases in dopamine D_2 receptor availability in the brain striatum and allowed the system to improve cognitive functioning. Fusar-Poli and colleagues[82] found gray matter volume decreases on MRI in people with schizophrenia were inversely correlated with cumulative exposure to antipsychotic treatments, whereas no effects were observed for duration of illness or illness severity.

In light of such concerns, several investigators have proposed that patients who have been stably maintained on antipsychotic medications should be given a trial to gradually taper or discontinue medications.[83] A review by Suzuki and Uchida[84] identified a subgroup of OAS who need little or no medication, either because symptoms had been stable or it was ineffective. Graff-Guerrero and colleagues'[85] study of OAS ages 50 and over found antipsychotic dose reduction was feasible in patients with stable illness and was accompanied by diminished adverse effects and improved illness severity measures. From a clinical standpoint, the therapeutic window of dopamine $D_{2/3}$ receptor occupancy in OAS (50%-60%) was lower than reported results for younger patients (65%–80%).

Because many persons with schizophrenia, especially early-onset cases, do not make full recoveries with medication regimens alone, a variety of nonpharmacological strategies have been devised specifically for older patients. Nonpharmacological approaches have focused on enhancing social cognition and perception, verbal communication, social skills, and interpersonal problem-solving skills. Randomized controlled studies have been conducted on 3 programs that have targeted middle-aged and older adults: functional adaptation skills training,[86] skills training combined with integrated care,[87] and cognitive behavioral social skills training.[88]

SUMMARY

- Point prevalence data indicate that approximately half of OAS are in clinical remission and one-quarter achieve community integration concomitantly with clinical remission. Longitudinally, persistent remission is less common (one-fourth) and the persistence of both remission and community integration is infrequent (one-eighth). Only 2% attain successful aging, that is, positive aging.
- For many persons, recovery continues into later life and is an ongoing process in which some persons improve with respect to remission and/or social integration and some worsen over time. For approximately two-fifths of persons who experience flux in these outcome categories, the notion that later life is a quiescent or stable end stage does not apply.
- There is some evidence that the accelerated aging model needs to be modified for OAS. The data have been mixed with respect to the prevalence of physical illness versus their age peers (although treatment rates may be lower), which may reflect a survivor effect. As many as fourth-fifths remained cognitively stable or improved over a 52-month follow-up interval. On the other hand, there is some support for higher levels of aging biomarkers.
- The paradoxic aging model, which overlaps to some extent with the accelerated aging model, also may require modification with respect to not only the physical and cognitive features but also psychosocial aspects. Again, there are

heterogeneous outcomes so that some persons show improvement in life quality and social integration, some show declines, and most remain stable over time.

- A dimensional model may be better for understanding depression and cognitive impairment in OAS. Although many persons have high levels of depression and cognitive deficits, they do not typically meet criteria of major depression nor do their cognitive deficits follow the typical patterns of AD.
- There are clinical and physiologic reasons to suggest that doses of antipsychotic medications can be reduced or, in some instances, eliminated. There are also nonpharmacological approaches that focus on improving social skills and social cognition that can complement features of the disorder that are not ameliorated by medication.
- Worldwide, the number of OAS continues to grow dramatically; however, only 1% of schizophrenia research has been devoted to this population.

REFERENCES

1. Laursen TM. Life expectancy among persons with schizophrenia or bipolar affective disorder. Schizophr Res 2011;131(1–3):101–4.
2. Jeste DV, Lanouette NM, Vahia IV. Schizophrenia and paranoid disorders. In: Blazer DG, Steffens DC, editors. Textbook of Geriatric Psychiatry. 4th edition. Washington, DC: American Psychiatric Publishing; 2009.
3. Meesters PD, de Haan L, Comijs HC, et al. Schizophrenia spectrum disorders in later life: prevalence and distribution of age at onset and sex in a Dutch catchment area. Am J Geriatr Psychiatry 2012;20(1):18–28.
4. Vahia IV, Cohen CI. Pychiatric disorders in later life. Schizophrenia and delusional disorders. In: Sadock BJ, Sadock VA, editors. Kaplan and Sadock's Comprehensive Textbook of Psychiatry. Philadelphia: Lippincott Williams & Wilkins; 2017.
5. Howard R, Rabins PV, Seeman MV, et al. Late-onset schizophrenia and very-late-onset schizophrenia-like psychosis: an international consensus. The International Late-Onset Schizophrenia Group. Am J Psychiatry 2000;157(2):172–8.
6. Vahia IV, Palmer BW, Depp C, et al. Is late-onset schizophrenia a subtype of schizophrenia? Acta Psychiatr Scand 2010;122(5):414–26.
7. Talaslahti T, Alanen HM, Hakko H, et al. Patients with very-late-onset schizophrenia-like psychosis have higher mortality rates than elderly patients with earlier onset schizophrenia. Int J Geriatr Psychiatry 2015;30(5):453–9.
8. Maglione JE, Vahia IV, Jeste DV. Schizophrenia spectrum and other psychotic disorders. In: Steffens DC, Blazer DG, Thakur ME, editors. Textbook of Geriatric Psychiatry. 5th edition. Washington, DC: American Psychiaitric Publishing; 2015.
9. Cohen CI, Vahia I, Reyes P, et al. Focus on geriatric psychiatry: schizophrenia in later life: clinical symptoms and social well-being. Psychiatr Serv 2008;59(3):232–4.
10. Cohen CI, Meesters PD, Zhao J. New perspectives on schizophrenia in later life: implications for treatment, policy, and research. Lancet Psychiatry 2015;2(4):340–50.
11. Keefe RS, Frescka E, Apter SH, et al. Clinical characteristics of Kraepelinian schizophrenia: replication and extension of previous findings. Am J Psychiatry 1996;153(6):806–11.
12. Substance Abuse and Mental Health Services Administration. SAMHSA's working definition of recovery. 10 guiding principles of recovery. *PEP12-RECDEF.* 2012.
13. Hegarty JD, Baldessarini RJ, Tohen M, et al. One hundred years of schizophrenia: a meta-analysis of the outcome literature. Am J Psychiatry 1994;151(10):1409–16.
14. American Psychiatric Association. Diagnostic and statistical manual of mental disorders. 3rd edition. Washington, DC: American Psychiatric Association; 1980.

15. Andreasen NC, Carpenter WT Jr, Kane JM, et al. Remission in schizophrenia: proposed criteria and rationale for consensus. Am J Psychiatry 2005;162(3):441–9.

16. Bankole A, Cohen CI, Vahia I, et al. Symptomatic remission in a multiracial urban population of older adults with schizophrenia. Am J Geriatr Psychiatry 2008; 16(12):966–73.

17. Leung WW, Bowie CR, Harvey PD. Functional implications of neuropsychological normality and symptom remission in older outpatients diagnosed with schizophrenia: a cross-sectional study. J Int Neuropsychol Soc 2008;14(3):479–88.

18. Meesters PD, Comijs HC, de Haan L, et al. Symptomatic remission and associated factors in a catchment area based population of older patients with schizophrenia. Schizophr Res 2011;126(1):237–44.

19. Harrison G, Hopper K, Craig T, et al. Recovery from psychotic illness: a 15- and 25-year international follow-up study. Br J Psychiatry 2001;178:506–17.

20. Cohen CI, Iqbal M. Longitudinal study of remission among older adults with schizophrenia spectrum disorder. Am J Geriatr Psychiatry 2014;22(5):450–8.

21. Won YL, Solomon PL. Community integration of persons with psychiatric disabilities in supportive independent housing: a conceptual model and methodological considerations. Ment Health Serv Res 2002;4(1):13–28.

22. Abdallah C, Cohen CI, Sanchez-Almira M, et al. Community integration and associated factors among older adults with schizophrenia. Psychiatr Serv 2009; 60(12):1642–8.

23. Jimenez C, Ryu HH, Garcia-Aracena E, et al. Community integration in older adults with schizophrenia on 4-year follow-up. American Journal of Geriatric Psychiatry 2012;20(3 suppl 1):S91.

24. Meesters PD, Stek ML, Comijs HC, et al. Social functioning among older community-dwelling patients with schizophrenia: a review. Am J Geriatr Psychiatry 2010;18(10):862–78.

25. Ibrahim F, Cohen CI, Ramirez PM. Successful aging in older adults with schizophrenia: prevalence and associated factors. Am J Geriatr Psychiatry 2010; 18(10):879–86.

26. Depp CA, Jeste DV. Definitions and predictors of successful aging: a comprehensive review of larger quantitative studies. Am J Geriatr Psychiatry 2006; 14(1):6–20.

27. Cohen CI, Talavera N, Hartung R. Depression among aging persons with schizophrenia who live in the community. Psychiatr Serv 1996;47(6):601–7.

28. Zisook S, McAdams LA, Kuck J, et al. Depressive symptoms in schizophrenia. Am J Psychiatry 1999;156(11):1736–43.

29. Jin H, Zisook S, Palmer BW, et al. Association of depressive symptoms with worse functioning in schizophrenia: a study in older outpatients. J Clin Psychiatry 2001; 62(10):797–803.

30. Diwan S, Cohen CI, Bankole AO, et al. Depression in older adults with schizophrenia spectrum disorders: prevalence and associated factors. Am J Geriatr Psychiatry 2007;15(12):991–8.

31. Zisook S, Montross L, Kasckow J, et al. Subsyndromal depressive symptoms in middle-aged and older persons with schizophrenia. Am J Geriatr Psychiatry 2007;15(12):1005–14.

32. Meesters PD, Comijs HC, Sonnenberg CM, et al. Prevalence and correlates of depressive symptoms in a catchment-area based cohort of older community-living schizophrenia patients. Schizophr Res 2014;157(1):285–91.

33. Kasckow J, Montross L, Prunty L, et al. Suicidal behavior in the older patient with schizophrenia. Aging Health 2011;7(3):379–93.

34. Cohen CI, Abdallah CG, Diwan S. Suicide attempts and associated factors in older adults with schizophrenia. Schizophr Res 2010;119(1):253–7.

35. Cohen CI, Ryu HH. A longitudinal study of the outcome and associated factors of subsyndromal and syndromal depression in community-dwelling older adults with schizophrenia spectrum disorder. Am J Geriatr Psychiatry 2015;23(9): 925–33.

36. Belitsky R, McGlashan TH. The manifestations of schizophrenia in late life: a dearth of data. Schizophr Bull 1993;19(4):683–5.

37. Ciompi L. Catamnestic long-term study on the course of life and aging of schizophrenics. Schizophr Bull 1980;6(4):606–18.

38. Cohen CI. Editorial comment: schizoaffective disorder in later life: "beware the Jabberwock". Am J Geriatr Psychiatry 2017;25(9):951–2.

39. Jeste DV, Wolkowitz OM, Palmer BW. Divergent trajectories of physical, cognitive, and psychosocial aging in schizophrenia. Schizophr Bull 2011;37(3):451–5.

40. Kirkpatrick B, Messias E, Harvey PD, et al. Is schizophrenia a syndrome of accelerated aging? Schizophr Bull 2008;34(6):1024–32.

41. Tsoutsoulas C, Mulsant BH, Kalache SM, et al. The influence of medical burden severity and cognition on functional competence in older community-dwelling individuals with schizophrenia. Schizophr Res 2016;170(2–3):330–5.

42. Rajji TK, Voineskos AN, Butters MA, et al. Cognitive performance of individuals with schizophrenia across seven decades: a study using the MATRICS consensus cognitive battery. Am J Geriatr Psychiatry 2013;21(2):108–18.

43. Savla GN, Moore DJ, Roesch SC, et al. An evaluation of longitudinal neurocognitive performance among middle-aged and older schizophrenia patients: use of mixed-model analyses. Schizophr Res 2006;83(2):215–23.

44. Murante T, Cohen CI. Cognitive functioning in older adults with schizophrenia. Focus 2017;15(1):26–34.

45. Kalache SM, Mulsant BH, Davies SJ, et al. The impact of aging, cognition, and symptoms on functional competence in individuals with schizophrenia across the lifespan. Schizophr Bull 2015;41(2):374–81.

46. Hendrie HC, Tu W, Tabbey R, et al. Health outcomes and cost of care among older adults with schizophrenia: a 10-year study using medical records across the continuum of care. Am J Geriatr Psychiatry 2014;22(5):427–36.

47. Ribe AR, Laursen TM, Charles M, et al. Long-term risk of dementia in persons with schizophrenia: a Danish population-based cohort study. JAMA Psychiatry 2015;72(11):1095–101.

48. Shah JN, Qureshi SU, Jawaid A, et al. Is there evidence for late cognitive decline in chronic schizophrenia? Psychiatr Q 2012;83(2):127–44.

49. Friedman JI, Harvey PD, Coleman T, et al. Six-year follow-up study of cognitive and functional status across the lifespan in schizophrenia: a comparison with Alzheimer's disease and normal aging. Am J Psychiatry 2001;158(9):1441–8.

50. Rajji TK, Ismail Z, Mulsant BH. Age at onset and cognition in schizophrenia: meta-analysis. Br J Psychiatry 2009;195(4):286–93.

51. Saha S, Chant D, McGrath J. A systematic review of mortality in schizophrenia: is the differential mortality gap worsening over time? Arch Gen Psychiatry 2007; 64(10):1123–31.

52. Talaslahti T, Alanen HM, Hakko H, et al. Mortality and causes of death in older patients with schizophrenia. Int J Geriatr Psychiatry 2012;27(11):1131–7.

53. Almeida OP, Hankey GJ, Yeap BB, et al. Mortality among people with severe mental disorders who reach old age: a longitudinal study of a community-representative sample of 37,892 men. PLoS One 2014;9(10):e111882.

54. Kredentser MS, Martens PJ, Chochinov HM, et al. Cause and rate of death in people with schizophrenia across the lifespan: a population-based study in Manitoba, Canada. J Clin Psychiatry 2014;75(2):154–61.

55. Vahia IV, Diwan S, Bankole AO, et al. Adequacy of medical treatment among older persons with schizophrenia. Psychiatr Serv 2008;59(8):853–9.

56. Brink M, Green A, Bojesen AB, et al. Physical health, medication, and healthcare utilization among 70-year-old people with schizophrenia: a nationwide Danish register study. Am J Geriatr Psychiatry 2017;25(5):500–9.

57. Stein-Parbury J, Gallagher R, Chenoweth L, et al. Factors associated with good self-management in older adults with a schizophrenic disorder compared with older adults with physical illnesses. J Psychiatr Ment Health Nurs 2012;19(2): 146–53.

58. Nguyen TT, Eyler LT, Jeste DV, et al. Systemic biomarkers of accelerated aging in schizophrenia: a critical review and future directions. Schizophrenia Bulletin, sbx069. https://doi.org/10.1093/schbul/sbx069.

59. Shepherd AM, Laurens KR, Matheson SL, et al. Systematic meta-review and quality assessment of the structural brain alterations in schizophrenia. Neurosci Biobehav Rev 2012;36(4):1342–56.

60. Heilbronner U, Samara M, Leucht S, et al. The longitudinal course of schizophrenia across the lifespan: clinical, cognitive, and neurobiological aspects. Harv Rev Psychiatry 2016;24(2):118.

61. Schnack HG, van Haren NE, Nieuwenhuis M, et al. Accelerated brain aging in schizophrenia: a longitudinal pattern recognition study. Am J Psychiatry 2016; 173(6):607–16.

62. Hahn C, Lim HK, Lee CU. Neuroimaging findings in late-onset schizophrenia and bipolar disorder. J Geriatr Psychiatry Neurol 2014;27(1):56–62.

63. Meesters PD, Comijs HC, de Haan L, et al. Subjective quality of life and its determinants in a catchment area based population of elderly schizophrenia patients. Schizophr Res 2013;147(2):275–80.

64. Cohen CI, Vengassery A, Garcia Aracena EF. A longitudinal analysis of quality of life and associated factors in older adults with schizophrenia spectrum disorder. Am J Geriatr Psychiatry 2017;25(7):755–65.

65. Bleuler M. Some results of research in schizophrenia. Behav Sci 1970;15(3): 211–9.

66. Shepherd S, Depp CA, Harris G, et al. Perspectives on schizophrenia over the lifespan: a qualitative study. Schizophr Bull 2012;38(2):295–303.

67. Martinsson G, Fagerberg I, Lindholm C, et al. Struggling for existence-Life situation experiences of older persons with mental disorders. Int J Qual Stud Health Well-being 2012. [Epub ahead of print].

68. Avieli H, Mushkin P, Araten-Bergman T, et al. Aging with schizophrenia: a lifelong experience of multidimensional losses and suffering. Arch Psychiatr Nurs 2016; 30(2):230–6.

69. Cohen CI, Hassamal SK, Begum N. General coping strategies and their impact on quality of life in older adults with schizophrenia. Schizophr Res 2011; 127(1–3):223–8.

70. Cohen CI. Age-related correlations in patient symptom management strategies in schizophrenia: an exploratory study. Int J Geriatr Psychiatry 1993;8(3):211–3.

71. Solano NH, Whitbourne SK. Coping with schizophrenia: patterns in later adulthood. Int J Aging Hum Dev 2001;53(1):1–10.

72. Cohen CI, Izediuno I, Yadack AM, et al. Characteristics of auditory hallucinations and associated factors in older adults with schizophrenia. Am J Geriatr Psychiatry 2014;22(5):442–9.

73. Essali A, Ali G. Antipsychotic drug treatment for elderly people with late-onset schizophrenia. Cochrane Database Syst Rev 2012;(2):CD004162.

74. Khan AY, Redden W, Ovais M, et al. Current concepts in the diagnosis and treatment of schizophrenia in later life. Curr Geriatr Rep 2015;4(4):290–300.

75. Alexopoulos GS, Streim J, Carpenter D, et al. Using antipsychotic agents in older patients. J Clin Psychiatry 2004;65(Suppl 2):5–99 [discussion: 100–2; quiz: 103–4].

76. Kulkarni J, Gavrilidis E, Gwini SM, et al. Effect of adjunctive raloxifene therapy on severity of refractory schizophrenia in women: a randomized clinical trial. JAMA Psychiatry 2016;73(9):947–54.

77. Usall J, Huerta-Ramos E, Labad J, et al. Raloxifene as an adjunctive treatment for postmenopausal women with schizophrenia: a 24-week double-blind, randomized, parallel, placebo-controlled trial. Schizophr Bull 2016;42(2):309–17.

78. Zisook S, Kasckow JW, Golshan S, et al. Citalopram augmentation for subsyndromal symptoms of depression in middle-aged and older outpatients with schizophrenia and schizoaffective disorder: a randomized controlled trial. J Clin Psychiatry 2009;70(4):562–71.

79. Liu AY, Rajji TK, Blumberger DM, et al. Brain stimulation in the treatment of late-life severe mental illness other than unipolar nonpsychotic depression. Am J Geriatr Psychiatry 2014;22(3):216–40.

80. Husa AP, Moilanen J, Murray GK, et al. Lifetime antipsychotic medication and cognitive performance in schizophrenia at age 43 years in a general population birth cohort. Psychiatry Res 2017;247:130–8.

81. Rajji TK, Mulsant BH, Nakajima S, et al. Cognition and dopamine D2 receptor availability in the striatum in older patients with schizophrenia. Am J Geriatr Psychiatry 2017;25(1):1–10.

82. Fusar-Poli P, Smieskova R, Kempton M, et al. Progressive brain changes in schizophrenia related to antipsychotic treatment? A meta-analysis of longitudinal MRI studies. Neurosci Biobehav Rev 2013;37(8):1680–91.

83. Jeste DV, Maglione JE. Treating older adults with schizophrenia: challenges and opportunities. Schizophr Bull 2013;39(5):966–8.

84. Suzuki T, Uchida H. Successful withdrawal from antipsychotic treatment in elderly male inpatients with schizophrenia–description of four cases and review of the literature. Psychiatry Res 2014;220(1–2):152–7.

85. Graff-Guerrero A, Rajji TK, Mulsant BH, et al. Evaluation of antipsychotic dose reduction in late-life schizophrenia: a prospective dopamine D2/3 receptor occupancy study. JAMA Psychiatry 2015;72(9):927–34.

86. Patterson TL, McKibbin C, Taylor M, et al. Functional adaptation skills training (FAST): a pilot psychosocial intervention study in middle-aged and older patients with chronic psychotic disorders. Am J Geriatr Psychiatry 2003;11(1):17–23.

87. Bartels SJ, Pratt SI, Mueser KT, et al. Long-term outcomes of a randomized trial of integrated skills training and preventive healthcare for older adults with serious mental illness. Am J Geriatr Psychiatry 2014;22(11):1251–61.

88. Granholm E, McQuaid JR, McClure FS, et al. A randomized, controlled trial of cognitive behavioral social skills training for middle-aged and older outpatients with chronic schizophrenia. Am J Psychiatry 2005;162(3):520–9.

Anxiety Disorders in Late Life

Katherine Ramos, PhD[a],*, Melinda A. Stanley, PhD[b]

KEYWORDS

- Late-life anxiety • Interventions
- Psychosocial and pharmacologic treatments for late-life anxiety • Older adults
- Mental health

KEY POINTS

- Research on late-life anxiety is a new but growing field.
- Pharmacotherapy and psychotherapy, or a combination, are viable anxiety treatments for older adults.
- Modifications and innovations to mental health treatments (eg, modular cognitive behavioral therapy, mindfulness, and acceptance therapies) offer enhanced opportunities to meet the needs of heterogeneous aging populations.

INTRODUCTION

The study of anxiety disorders in later life is a relatively new field representing some of the most significant mental health problems affecting older adults. Prevalence estimates of anxiety disorders in late life vary considerably based on multiple methodological issues (eg, sampling strategies, cut-off score to define older adults), and current diagnostic criteria may not adequately capture the nature and experience of anxiety in older people, particularly those in ethnic and racial minority groups. Current estimates, however, suggest 1-year prevalence up to 11.6% for older adults in the United States[1] and lifetime prevalence as high as 15.1%.[2] Prevalence in other countries ranges from 4.4% to 14.2%.[3] Across all epidemiologic surveys to date, anxiety disorders are more common in later life than depression.

Among older adults, anxiety disorders and subsyndromal anxiety are associated with increased physical disability,[4] increased risk for cognitive impairment and dementia,[5] poorer quality of life, and increased health service use.[6] Longitudinal studies

Disclosure Statement: K. Ramos and M.A. Stanley have nothing to disclose.
[a] Geriatric, Education, Research and Clinical Center (GRECC), Durham VA Medical Center, 508 Fulton Street (GRECC 182), Durham, NC 27705, USA; [b] Baylor College of Medicine, Center for Innovations in Quality, Effectiveness and Safety, Michael E. DeBakey VA Medical Center, (MEDVAMC 152), 2002 Holcombe Boulevard, Houston, TX 77030, USA
* Corresponding author.
E-mail address: Katherine.ramos@va.gov

Psychiatr Clin N Am 41 (2018) 55–64
https://doi.org/10.1016/j.psc.2017.10.005
0193-953X/18/Published by Elsevier Inc.

psych.theclinics.com

show persistence of anxiety over time, high relapse rates, and significant increased risk of depression.[7] Clearly, the personal and public health impact of late-life anxiety is remarkable and requires continued clinical and scientific attention.

This article reviews late-life anxiety disorders using recent classifications in the *Diagnostic and Statistical Manual of Mental Disorders* (DSM), 5th edition,[8] with attention to generalized anxiety disorder (GAD), social anxiety disorder, specific phobias (eg, fear of falling), and panic disorder. Pharmacologic and psychotherapy approaches to treat late-life anxiety are reviewed with special attention to innovations in clinical care across settings, treatment models, and treatment delivery.

PREVALENCE AND NATURE OF ANXIETY DISORDERS IN LATER LIFE
Generalized Anxiety Disorder

GAD is among the most common of the anxiety disorders in older adults, with 6-month and 12-month prevalence ranging from 1.2% to 7.3%,[3] and lifetime prevalence as high as 11%.[9] The disorder is even more common among people with chronic illness (19%)[10]; however, GAD in later life is frequently unrecognized and untreated.[11]

Recognizing GAD among older adults is particularly difficult given that associated physical symptoms (eg, sleep disturbance, fatigue, restlessness, and difficulty concentrating) overlap significantly with symptoms of normal aging, medical conditions, and medications commonly used in later life. Older adults infrequently use psychological terms to describe anxiety (eg, concerns, fret, or think too much vs worry or anxiety) and they are less able than younger adults to identify accurately the symptoms of anxiety.[12]

Worry content among older adults typically reflects problems that arise in later stages of life (eg, health, welfare or loss of loved ones, life transitions, retirement, caregiving responsibilities), and economic and legal issues (eg, reduced income, increased health care costs, end-of-life planning). GAD onset, however, seems to have a bimodal distribution, with substantial numbers of people reporting symptoms since late adolescence or early adulthood and others indicating more recent onset (eg, after age 50 years).[3] Risk factors for late-onset GAD include gender (female), adverse life events, and chronic physical or mental health disorders.[13] Early-onset GAD is associated with greater symptom severity and increased mental health comorbidity but also reduced health-related quality of life.[3]

Specific Phobias and Fear of Falling

Community prevalence of specific phobias among older adults ranges from 3.1% (6-month) to 10.1% (current), although in some cases other diagnoses (eg, agoraphobia) or remitted diagnoses are counted, artificially inflating published rates.[3] Older people with specific fears also sometimes fail to recognize or acknowledge the excessiveness of these fears, leading to high rates of subthreshold phobias that are associated with increased chronic health problems and coexistent depression comparable to what is observed in DSM-specific phobia.[14]

The most common specific fear among older people is fear of falling. This fear is not addressed specifically in DSM-5; however, prevalence among older adults ranges from 12% to 65%, with even higher rates among people with a history of falls (92%).[15] Fear of falling is linked to reduced self-efficacy for managing falls and lower balance confidence, and prevalence increases with age. Considerable impairment can result given associated withdrawal from physical and social activities, although, as with other specific phobias, failure to recognize fear of falling as a condition in need of treatment is often related to older adults' failure to recognize the excessiveness of their fears.

Social Anxiety Disorder and Panic Disorder

Prevalence of social anxiety disorder (social phobia) in later life is between .6% (12-month) and 6.6% (lifetime).[3] As with other specific phobias, onset is typically not in later life and projected prevalence may be underestimated given older adults' tendencies not to recognize excessiveness of fear. Coexistent depression is common, as are other anxiety disorders, and the presence of these disorders significantly affects overall functional status and health-related quality of life.[16]

Panic disorder is relatively infrequent in older adults, with 6-month and 12-month prevalence of 1.0% or lower and lifetime rates up to 2.0%.[3] Onset is typically in younger adulthood. Older adults with panic disorder (age 60 years or more) have fewer panic symptoms, better global functioning, and less severe comorbid depressive symptoms than younger adults with the disorder, although rates of coexistent psychiatric disorders are comparable.[17] Age of onset seems to have little association with panic disorder severity and impact.

Special Populations

Diverse aging adults

Women and racial and ethnic minorities make up the fastest growing segment of the elderly population. Anxiety disorders in later life are more common among women.[3] Although inadequate diagnostic criteria may artificially reduce available prevalence estimates, non-Hispanic white people and Latinos have the highest rates of anxiety disorders.[18] High rates of GAD have been reported among African American women (3.7%) and very low rates among African American men (0.3%).[19] Poverty, parental loss or separation, and low affective support also are associated with the incidence of GAD among older adults.[9]

Neurocognitive disease

Prevalence of anxiety disorders among people with neurocognitive disorder (NCD) range from 5% to 21%, and up to 71% have significant anxiety symptoms.[20] Identifying anxiety in people with neurocognitive impairment is complicated; however, comorbid anxiety and NCD are associated with reduced quality of life, restlessness, increased functional limitations, poorer physical health, and increased rate of nursing home placement.[20] Some data also suggest an increased rate (up to 5 times more likely) of conversion from mild NCD to major NCD when anxiety symptoms are present.[3]

Chronic health and multimorbidity

Up to 92% of older adults have at least 1 chronic medical condition and approximately 40% have multimorbidity, defined as 3 or more of these conditions.[21] Anxiety disorders are more common among people suffering from chronic medical disease, and the number of medical illnesses is positively associated with the presence of anxiety. Multimorbidity, in fact, confers a 2.3-fold increase in the occurrence of anxiety.[21] Cardiovascular disease, hyperthyroidism, arthritis and chronic pain, Parkinson disease, diabetes, high blood pressure, lung disease, and gastrointestinal (GI) problems are all associated with increased rates of anxiety,[15,21] and complicated reciprocal relations of medical and anxiety symptoms create difficulties for diagnosis.

Anxiety is also prevalent among older adults receiving palliative and hospice care. In palliative care settings, prevalence of anxiety can be as high as 25%.[22] Common etiologic factors include preexisting anxiety, continued advancement of progressive or terminal illness, medications (eg, psychostimulants or rapid discontinuation of opiates), and fear of dying.[22] Anxiety treatment in geriatric palliative care is complicated given cooccurring medical complexities, uncertainty about disease prognosis, and sustained worry about how illness may affect financial, personal, and social circumstances.

OVERVIEW OF LATE-LIFE ANXIETY TREATMENTS
Medication

Benzodiazepines remain the most frequently prescribed medications for late-life anxiety.[3] Short-term, positive effects of these medications make them an attractive option for both prescribers and patients, and prescription rates are even higher for older people than for younger adults.[23] However, use of benzodiazepines among older adults creates significant increased risk of serious adverse events, including falls, psychomotor functioning, cognitive decline, disability, and motor vehicle accidents.[15] As such, these and other medications with sedative effects (eg, anticholinergic, antihistaminergic) should be used only as short-term adjuncts to treatment, although some experts recommend avoiding these medications whenever possible.[15]

First-line medications for late-life anxiety include the selective serotonergic reuptake inhibitors (SSRIs) and the serotonin-norepinephrine reuptake inhibitors (SNRIs). A handful of clinical trials have demonstrated positive effects relative to placebo for citalopram, escitalopram, paroxetine, sertraline, venlafaxine, and duloxetine.[3,15] Most of these trials have focused on treatment outcomes for older adults with GAD; however, positive effects also have been demonstrated for late-life panic disorder and in mixed samples. Although these medications are generally well-tolerated among older adults, adverse effect profiles require increased attention to potential gait impairment and non-GI and GI bleeding, relative to younger adults.[15]

Psychosocial Treatments

Research on evidence-based psychosocial treatments for late-life anxiety is growing (**Box 1**). In the last 10 years, meta-analytic research and independent studies support the efficacy of cognitive behavioral treatment (CBT) for late-life GAD.[24] Two recent meta-analyses also support the use of CBT for symptom reduction across a wide range of late-life anxiety disorders, including GAD, panic disorder, mixed anxiety disorders, and anxiety symptoms when compared with treatment as usual, control, or waitlist conditions.[25] Effects of CBT are small relative to alternative active treatments, in particular, supportive therapy.

CBT also is effective when compared with paroxetine and waitlist control groups.[26] Effects of CBT on panic symptoms are comparable for younger and older adults, with moderate to large effect sizes, although slightly higher improvements in avoidance behavior occur among older adults.[27] However, despite the efficacy of CBT for late-

---

Box 1
Evidence-based treatments for late-life anxiety

- Cognitive behavioral therapy is a short-term, goal-oriented treatment designed to reduce anxiety symptoms by modifying maladaptive behavior and patterns of thinking about the self, others, or the world.

- Relaxation training teaches techniques to reduce physical symptoms of anxiety or stress. Examples include progressive muscle relaxation, deep breathing, and visual guided imagery.

- Supportive therapy provides psychological support to help clients manage anxiety or distress via active listening, encouragement, offering comfort, and empathic understanding.

life anxiety, effects remain small when compared with active treatments (eg, supportive therapy) and results are not as robust as in younger adult populations.

There are, however, limitations to psychosocial treatments. Specifically, initial efficacy trials included samples that were homogeneous regarding diagnosis and demographic characteristics. Additionally, most studies were conducted in academic clinical settings, limiting generalizability about treatment efficacy and outcomes. The complexity for older adults to access and receive treatment has led to innovations across treatment settings, treatment modifications for evidence-based psychosocial treatments, and innovative delivery options to enhance outcomes and engagement. Treatment modifications align with the Institute of Medicine's (2012) mission to improve health service delivery that emphasizes comprehensive, interdisciplinary, and patient-centered care.[28]

CLINICAL CARE INNOVATIONS
Innovations Across Settings

The provision of mental health care can be improved by treatment dissemination efforts across nontraditional settings. By and large, most evidence-based treatments are delivered in tightly controlled research settings. However, incorporating treatments into medical settings, home-based care, and the community may improve opportunities to increase treatment engagement for older adults. In general, integrating behavioral health services in nontraditional mental health settings with further inclusion of a larger and diverse interdisciplinary workforce can yield improved outcomes and reduce costs in care.[28]

Primary care

Primary care continues to be the most common setting in which older adults are screened, diagnosed, and treated for late-life anxiety. Although rates of anxiety disorders in primary care are high,[29] and most older adults (up to 73%) rely on primary care services to receive mental health treatment, late-life anxiety is often underrecognized and poorly treated in this setting.[30] In the United States, new integrated models of care for late-life anxiety have been tested in primary care settings with positive outcomes. In particular, 2 large randomized clinical trials have demonstrated the effectiveness of CBT-based treatment of late-life GAD delivered in primary care.[31,32] In both trials, treatment included a combination of skills-based sessions and follow-up booster calls. Effects were positive for worry or GAD severity, depression, and general mental health.

Increased attention to mental health service delivery in primary care has many benefits, including so-called warm-hand-offs, same-day visits, and increased treatment engagement. However, translating evidence-based treatments into primary care may not always be feasible under circumstances in which expert providers are unavailable, poor infrastructure exists for implementing services, and financial costs to sustain implementation efforts become unwieldly. Future studies need to emphasize the development of implementation strategies, policy, and infrastructure changes to support new models of care delivery.[28,33]

Home-based care and community settings

In the United States, 9.2% of 40 million older adults meet criteria for needing home-based care.[34] The prevalence of depression and anxiety disorders almost doubles for those managing medical complexities or experiencing cognitive impairment.[35] Untreated mental health symptoms among this population negatively impact medical, social, and functional abilities, driving overuse of health care (as high as 70% among low income older adults).[36]

To date, most home-based mental health care has demonstrated success in the treatment of depression in older adults.[37,38] Examples are the Program to Encourage Active, Rewarding Lives for Seniors (PEARLS) and Healthy Identifying Depression, Empowering Activities for Seniors (Healthy IDEAS). In reported case studies, home-based care for late-life anxiety has shown positive outcomes for medically complex older adults with long histories of chronic mental health issues and limited access to social support.[39] Among older adults with mild or moderate dementia, a home-based cognitive behavioral intervention led to significant reductions in anxiety symptoms and caregiver distress at posttreatment, in addition to higher self-reported quality of life, compared with usual care.[40] Despite treatment feasibility, however, improvements in treatment outcomes were not maintained at 6-month follow-up.

Regarding community-based care, an initial pilot randomized trial of a modified version of CBT (Calmer Life, a person-centered, innovative modular intervention with opportunities for participants to include religious and spiritual values) incorporated resource counseling to addresses basic unmet needs in addition to enhanced communication with health care providers for underserved older adults.[41] Results of this pilot demonstrated reductions in worry, anxiety, and depression, as well as improved sleep and mental health quality of life relative to enhanced community care (ECC), which consists of standard community-based information and referral.[41] A larger trial of the Calmer Life intervention is ongoing in the context of a community-academic partnership with social service and faith-based organizations in low-income, predominantly African American communities that are underserved for mental health care access.[42] A Spanish-language version of the intervention, Vida Calma, was piloted and found feasible for use with an older adult participant who experienced improvements in symptoms of anxiety depression, and satisfaction with life.[43]

Innovations Across Mental Health Treatment Models

In addition to expanding settings in which EBPs are delivered, other modifications in treatment models have been developed to better meet the unique needs of older adults in real-world care. Noteworthy examples include person-centered, modular treatments with options for both in-person and telephone-based treatments.[32] Others have addressed cultural preferences (eg, inclusion of religious and spiritual preferences, language translations) and social service needs.[41–43] Other CBT-based interventions have also found success in improving symptoms of late-life anxiety with special attention to comorbid conditions such as neurocognitive difficulties[44] and chronic illness.[45]

Acceptance-based and mindfulness-based interventions

Although CBT is the most widely tested psychotherapy approach for late-life anxiety, this model of treatment alone may be insufficient in treating anxiety. Two alternative treatments, Acceptance and Commitment Therapy (ACT) and Mindfulness-Based Stress Reduction (MBSR), are innovative approaches that may be useful for older adults, specifically in the treatment of anxiety.[46] Like CBT, ACT and MBSR make use of behavioral skills that include diaphragmatic breathing and behavioral activation. ACT and MBSR emphasize psychological flexibility by helping individuals better adapt to their individual experiences without attempting to change problematic behaviors or thoughts. These treatments may benefit older adults in finding acceptance toward life experiences that are nonmodifiable (eg, worsening health, shifts in gains and losses in older age).

Innovations in Delivery Options and Mental Health Workforce

A growing number of late-life anxiety studies have found positive outcomes following the delivery of telephone-based treatments, Internet-delivered treatments, and self-guided interventions. Some interventions offer flexible formats that include both telephone and in-person sessions, whereas other approaches use a single format. For example, telephone-based CBT (CBT-T) was more effective than an information-only control condition in reducing GAD symptoms, depression, and worry in older adults with GAD.[47] In a recent long-term follow-up, CBT-T for GAD compared with nondirective supportive therapy was superior in reducing late-life GAD 1 year after posttreatment completion.[48]

In another study, positive effects in symptom reduction for anxiety and/or depression were found with modular telephone CBT-T intervention (Veterans Affairs [VA] Home-based Emotional Learning with Practical Skills Program [VA-HELPS]) delivered to rural dwelling older adult veterans receiving home-based primary care.[49] Among the 3 case studies presented, older adult veterans varied in functional status, had 3 or more chronic health conditions, and reported moderate to severe symptoms of anxiety and depression. Participation in VA-HELPS offered personalized treatment tailored to patient needs with opportunities to incorporate religious and spiritual values and preferences. Posttreatment, participants showed improvements in depression and anxiety symptoms, suggesting that CBT-T in home care is an acceptable form of treatment of older adults experiencing late-life depression and/or anxiety symptoms.

In another trial, Internet-delivered, self-guided CBT was effective in reducing symptoms of anxiety and depression among older adults with self-reported clinically significant symptoms of GAD compared with a control group at posttreatment.[50] In this 8-week intervention, participants had access to 5 online sessions containing lesson summaries and homework assignments. Materials were made available as appropriate to reduce participants from moving through content material too quickly, with therapists making weekly (check in) calls lasting no more than 10 minutes. Symptom gains remained at 3-month and 12-month follow-up. Reductions in GAD have also been reported in self-guided CBT-T treatment with gains maintained over a 1-year period.[51]

Offering flexible delivery formats increases access and improves treatment engagement. However, the success of innovations in treatment and delivery will require an increased expansion of the geriatric workforce that extends beyond licensed mental health professionals.[28] Expansions may include training of nontraditional health care providers such as community health workers, social workers, case managers, and nurses. In fact, previous work has found that lay providers (ie, nonlicensed bachelor level providers) can effectively deliver CBT for older adults with late-life anxiety with outcomes comparable to PhD-level providers.[32] The Calmer Life intervention also follows a model of care with delivery by community providers.[42] Expanding training and supervision for nonlicensed providers has many advantages, including the opportunity to extend mental health services and reduce cost of service delivery by nearly 2-fold.[33]

SUMMARY

The study of late-life anxiety is a new yet highly promising field. Current evidence suggests that pharmacotherapy or psychotherapy, or a combination, are viable anxiety treatments for older adults. SSRIs and SNRIs have proven effective and pose as better alternatives to benzodiazepines given adverse effects that include fall risks, disability, and cognitive impairment. Use of psychosocial treatments, such as CBT, has also proven efficacious in treating anxiety and worry among older adults. However, more research is needed to address how service delivery can (1) be improved, (2) be offered in a variety of nontraditional mental health settings, and (3) meet the unique needs of heterogeneous aging populations. Innovations in treatment models (eg, modular CBT, mindfulness, and acceptance therapies) and flexible delivery formats are forward-thinking solutions that will benefit from further testing. Future studies that can mirror real-world care and place greater attention on social and cultural modifications while offering innovative solutions for implementation are promising and have important clinical care implications.

REFERENCES

1. Reynolds K, Pietrzak RH, El-Gabalawy R, et al. Prevalence of psychiatric disorders in US older adults: findings from a nationally representative survey. World Psychiatr 2015;14:74–81.
2. Kessler R, Berglund P, Demler O, et al. Lifetime prevalence and age-of-onset distributions of DSM-IV disorders in the national comorbidity survey replication. Arch Gen Psychiatry 2005;62(6):593–602.
3. Wolitzky-Taylor K, Castriotta N, Lenze E, et al. Anxiety disorders in older adults: a comprehensive review. Depress Anxiety 2010;27(2):190–211.
4. Brenes GA, Guralnik JM, Williamson JD, et al. The influence of anxiety on the progression of disability. J Am Geriatr Soc 2005;53(1):34–9.
5. Gulpers B, Ramakers I, Hamel R, et al. Anxiety as a predictor for cognitive decline and dementia: a systematic review and meta-analysis. Am J Geriatr Psychiatry 2016;24:823–42.
6. Porensky EK, Dew MA, Karp JF, et al. The burden of late-life generalized anxiety disorder: effects on disability, health-related quality of life, and healthcare utilization. Am J Geriatr Psychiatry 2009;17(6):473–82.
7. Sami MB, Nilforooshan R. The natural course of anxiety disorders in the elderly: a systematic review of longitudinal trials. Int Psychogeriatr 2015;27(7):1061–9.
8. American Psychiatric Association. Diagnostic and statistical manual of mental disorders (5th edition). Washington, DC: American Psychiatric Association; 2013.
9. Zhang X, Norton J, Carriere I, et al. Generalized anxiety in community-dwelling elderly: Prevalence and clinical characteristics. J Affect Disord 2015;172:24–9.
10. Kunik ME, Roundy K, Veazey C, et al. Surprisingly high prevalence of anxiety and depression in chronic breathing disorders. Chest 2005;127(4):1205–11.
11. Calleo J, Stanley MA, Greisinger A, et al. Generalized anxiety disorder in older medical patients: diagnostic recognition, mental health management and service utilization. J Clin Psychol Med Settings 2009;16:178–85.
12. Wetherell JL, Petkus AJ, McChesney K, et al. Older adults are less accurate than younger adults at identifying symptoms of anxiety and depression. J Nerv Ment Dis 2009;197(8):623–6.
13. Zhang X, Norton J, Carriere I, et al. Risk factors for late-onset generalized anxiety disorder: Results from a 12-year prospective cohort (The ESPRIT study). Transl Psychiatry 2015;5:1–7.
14. Grenier S, Schuurmans J, Goldfarb M, et al. The epidemiology of specific phobia and subthreshold fear subtypes in a community-based sample of older adults. Depress Anxiety 2011;28:456–63.
15. Bower ES, Wetherell JL, Mon T, et al. Treating anxiety disorders in older adults: current treatments and future directions. Harv Rev Psychiatry 2015;23:329–42.

16. Chou KL. Social anxiety disorder in older adults: Evidence from the National Epidemiologic Survey on alcohol and related conditions. J Affect Disord 2009; 119:76–83.

17. Sheikh JI, Swales PJ, Carlson EB, et al. Aging and panic disorder: phenomenology, comorbidity, and risk factors. Am J Geriatr Psychiatry 2004;12(1):102–9.

18. Jimenez DE, Alegría M, Chen CN, et al. Prevalence of psychiatric illnesses in older ethnic minority adults. J Am Geriatr Soc 2010;58(2):256–64.

19. Blazer DG, Hughes D, George LK, et al. Generalized anxiety disorder. In: Robbins LN, Regier DA, editors. Psychiatric disorders in America. 1st edition. New York: Free Press; 1991. p. 181–203.

20. Seignourel P, Kunik M, Snow L, et al. Anxiety in dementia: a critical review. Clin Psychol Rev 2008;28(7):1071–82.

21. Gould CE, O'Hara R, Goldstein MK, et al. Multimorbidity is associated with anxiety in older adults in the Health and Retirement Study. Int J Geriatr Psychiatry 2016;31(10):1105–15.

22. Chai E, Meier D, Morris J, et al, editors. Geriatric palliative care: a practical guide for clinicians. New York: Oxford University Press; 2014.

23. Conti EC, Stanley MA, Amspoker AB, et al. Sedative-hypnotic use among older adults participating in anxiety research. Int J Aging Hum Dev 2017;85:3–17.

24. Hall J, Kellett S, Berrios R, et al. Efficacy of cognitive behavioral therapy for generalized anxiety disorder in older adults: systematic review, meta-analysis, and meta-regression. Am J Geriatr Psychiatry 2016;24(11):1063–73.

25. Thorp SR, Ayers C, Nuevo R, et al. Meta-analysis comparing different behavioral treatments for late-life anxiety. Am J Geriatr Psychiatry 2009;17(2):105–15.

26. Hendriks G, Keijsers G, Kampman M, et al. Predictors of outcome of pharmacological and psychological treatment of late-life panic disorder with agoraphobia. Int J Geriatr Psychiatry 2012;27(2):146–50.

27. Hendriks G, Kampman M, Keijsers G, et al. Cognitive-behavioral therapy for panic disorder with agoraphobia in older people: a comparison with younger patients. Depress Anxiety 2014;31(8):669–77.

28. Institute of Medicine. Mental health and substance use workforce for older adults: in whose hands? Washington, DC: National Academy Press; 2012.

29. Kroenke K, Spitzer RL, Williams JB, et al. Anxiety disorders in primary care: Prevalence, impairment, comorbidity, and detection. Ann Intern Med 2007;146(5): 317–25.

30. Byers AL, Arean PA, Yaffe K. Low use of mental health services among older Americans with mood and anxiety disorders. Psychiatr Serv 2012;63(1):66–72.

31. Stanley MA, Wilson N, Novy D, et al. Cognitive behavior therapy for generalized anxiety disorder among older adults in primary care. J Am Med Assoc 2009; 301(14):1460–7.

32. Stanley MA, Wilson N, Amspoker A, et al. Lay providers can deliver effective cognitive behavior therapy for older adults with generalized anxiety disorder: a randomized trial. Depress Anxiety 2014;31(5):391–401.

33. Kunik ME, Mills WL, Amspoker AB, et al. Expanding the geriatric mental health workforce through utilization of non-licensed providers. Aging Ment Health 2016;1–7. https://doi.org/10.1080/13607863.2016.1186150.

34. Qiu WQ, Dean M, Liu T, et al. Physical and mental health of homebound older adults: an overlooked population. J Am Geriatr Soc 2010;58(12):2423–8.

35. Gellis ZD. Depression screening in medically ill homecare elderly. Best Pract Ment Health 2010;6(1):1–16.

36. Musich S, Wang SS, Hawkins K, et al. Homebound older adults: prevalence, characteristics, health care utilization and quality of care. Geriatr Nurs 2015; 36(6):445–50.
37. Ciechanowski P, Wagner E, Schmaling K, et al. Community-integrated home-based depression treatment in the elderly: a randomized controlled trial. J Am Med Assoc 2004;291:1569–77.
38. Quijano LM, Stanley MA, Petersen NJ, et al. Healthy IDEAS A depression intervention delivered by community-based case managers serving older adults. J Appl Gerontol 2007;26(2):139–56.
39. Diefenbach G, Tolin D, Gilliam C, et al. Extending cognitive-behavioral therapy for late-life anxiety to home care: Program development and case examples. Behav Modif 2008;32(5):595–610.
40. Stanley MA, Calleo J, Bush AL, et al. The peaceful mind program: a pilot test of a CBT-based intervention for anxious patients with dementia. Am J Geriatr Psychiatry 2013;21(7):696–708.
41. Stanley MA, Wilson N, Shrestha S, et al. Calmer life: a culturally tailored intervention for anxiety in underserved older adults. Am J Geriatr Psychiatry 2016;24(8): 648–58.
42. Shrestha S, Wilson N, Kunik ME, et al. Calmer life: a hybrid effectiveness-implementation trial for late-life anxiety conducted in low-income, mental health-underserved communities. J Psychiatr Pract 2017;23(3):180–90.
43. Ramos K, Cortes J, Wilson N, et al. Vida calma: CBT for anxiety with a Spanish-speaking Hispanic adult. Clin Gerontol 2017;40(3):213–9.
44. Calleo J, Amspoker A, Sarwar A, et al. A pilot study of a cognitive-behavioral treatment for anxiety and depression in patients with Parkinson disease. J Geriatr Psychiatry Neurol 2015;28(3):210–7.
45. Cully J, Stanley MA, Kauth MR, et al. Effectiveness and implementation of brief cognitive behavioral therapy in VA primary care settings. Unpublished poster presentation at the annual Health Services Research and Development/QUERI National Conference. Philadelphia (PA), July 8–10, 2015.
46. Wetherell JL, Afari N, Ayers C, et al. Acceptance and commitment therapy for generalized anxiety disorder in older adults: a preliminary report. Behav Ther 2011;42(1):127–34.
47. Brenes GA, Miller M, Williamson J, et al. A randomized controlled trial of telephone-delivered cognitive-behavioral therapy for late-life anxiety disorders. Am J Geriatr Psychiatry 2012;20(8):707–16.
48. Brenes GA, Danhauer SC, Lyles MF, et al. Long-term effects of telephone-delivered psychotherapy for late-life gad. Am J Geriatr Psychiatry 2017. https://doi.org/10.1016/j.jagp.2017.05.013.
49. Barrera TL, Cummings JP, Armento M, et al. Telephone-delivered cognitive-behavioral therapy for older, rural veterans with depression and anxiety in home-based primary care. Clin Gerontol 2017;40(2):114–23.
50. Dear BF, Zou JB, Ali S, et al. Clinical and cost-effectiveness of therapist-guided internet-delivered cognitive behavior therapy for older adults with symptoms of anxiety: a randomized controlled trial. Behav Ther 2015;46(2):206–17.
51. Landreville P, Gosselin P, Grenier S, et al. Guided self-help for generalized anxiety disorder in older adults. Aging Ment Health 2016;20(10):1070–83.

Evaluating Cognitive Reserve Through the Prism of Preclinical Alzheimer Disease

Anja Soldan, PhD*, Corinne Pettigrew, PhD, Marilyn Albert, PhD

KEYWORDS

- Cognitive reserve • Alzheimer disease • Mild cognitive impairment • Biomarkers
- Amyloid • Tau • Atrophy

KEY POINTS

- Evidence indicates that higher levels of cognitive reserve (CR), as measured by proxy variables such as educational and occupational attainment, delay the onset of symptoms of mild cognitive impairment due to Alzheimer disease.
- Recent findings suggest that the protective effects of CR may be independent of amyloid pathologic features but interact with measures of neuronal injury to alter risk of cognitive impairment.
- It is unclear whether CR alters future risk of cognitive decline by directly affecting brain pathologic features.
- Prospective longitudinal biomarker studies are needed to investigate the mechanisms by which CR alters future risk of cognitive decline.

OVERVIEW: THE CONCEPT OF COGNITIVE RESERVE

The aging of the population, which is accompanied by an increasing prevalence of AD, makes it imperative to identify factors that reduce risk of onset of dementia. CR is increasingly being studied as a potential mechanism for reducing the risk of cognitive decline and dementia among older adults. The concept of CR grew out of observations that there can be a marked discrepancy between an individual's clinical symptomatology and estimates of the amount of neuropathologic features in the brain. For example, an early study by Stern and colleagues[1] (1992) that began investigating this issue reported that among individuals with probable AD and matched for clinical

Disclosure: M. Albert is a consultant to Eli Lilly and has funding from Avid Radiopharmaceuticals. A. Soldan and C. Pettigrew have nothing to disclose. The preparation of this article was supported in part by grants from the National Institute on Aging: U19-AG03365, P50-AG005146.
Department of Neurology, Johns Hopkins School of Medicine, 1620 McElderry Street, Reed Hall West - 1, Baltimore, MD 21205, USA
* Corresponding author.
E-mail address: asoldan1@jhmi.edu

Psychiatr Clin N Am 41 (2018) 65–77
https://doi.org/10.1016/j.psc.2017.10.006
0193-953X/18/© 2017 Elsevier Inc. All rights reserved.

severity, those with more years of education had more advanced pathologic features, as indicated by less cerebral blood flow in AD-vulnerable regions.

It has been proposed that lifetime experiences that are associated with cognitive stimulation (eg, years of education, occupational attainment, and engagement in mentally stimulating leisure activities) modify the brain in a way that allows individuals to tolerate greater levels of neuropathologic features or injury before showing symptoms of functional decline.[2] Although the concept of CR has primarily been studied within the context of AD, it is hypothesized to apply to any brain disease or condition that results in brain damage, and an increasing number of studies support this proposal.[3–5] It has also been proposed that CR moderates the relationship between brain changes and age-related cognitive decline.[2,6]

This article first briefly summarizes the major lines of evidence in support of the concept of CR within the context of AD. It then provides a detailed review of longitudinal biomarker studies that have examined the relationship between measures of CR, AD pathologic features, and subsequent cognitive change or impairment among individuals who were cognitively normal when first evaluated. It focuses on studies of individuals with normal cognition at baseline because it is now recognized that AD pathologic features begin to develop when individuals are cognitively normal, a phase of the disease commonly referred to as preclinical AD.[7] As such, these types of studies provide insight into how and to what extent CR delays the onset of the symptomatic phase of the disease, which has major public health implications; it has been estimated that interventions that delay the onset of dementia by 5 years would reduce the prevalence of dementia by 50%.[8]

EVIDENCE IN SUPPORT OF COGNITIVE RESERVE

Supporting the concept of CR, many large prospective epidemiologic studies of initially nondemented individuals have shown that more years of education,[9] greater occupational breadth and complexity,[9,10] and greater lifetime engagement in cognitively stimulating activities[11] are associated with a reduced risk of dementia. The evidence regarding the relationship between measures of CR and rates of change in cognition is more mixed, with many recent studies reporting little or no association between CR and rates of cognitive decline, despite evidence that individuals with higher CR have a higher performance on cognitive tests.[12] It has been suggested that the differences in findings among these studies likely reflect methodological and cohort differences and, taken together, the evidence indicates that CR primarily influences baseline levels of cognitive performance.[12,13] Thus, epidemiologic studies strongly support the notion that higher levels of CR are associated with better cognitive performance, as well as a reduced risk of developing dementia later in life, whereas the impact of CR on the trajectory of cognitive decline is less clear. Epidemiologic research on CR, however, has generally been limited by a lack of measures of underlying AD pathologic features. As such, these types of studies cannot directly examine whether and how measures of CR affect the association between levels of neuropathologic features and cognitive performance.

Thus, studies that have incorporated biomarkers, which are considered an indirect reflection of underlying neuropathologic features, are of particular importance in clarifying the mechanisms by which CR may be protective. Most studies on CR with biomarker measures of AD pathologic features have been cross-sectional in nature. A common finding of cross-sectional studies is that, at similar levels of cognitive functioning, individuals with higher CR tend to have biomarker measures reflecting higher levels AD pathologic features in the brain. For example, atrophy measures based on

MRI,[14–16] and levels of amyloid and tau derived from PET imaging[17,18] or measured in cerebrospinal fluid (CSF),[19] tend to be more abnormal among individuals with higher CR. These findings suggest that the effects of AD pathologic features on cognition are reduced in individuals with higher reserve. Some cross-sectional studies also suggest that the effects of aging on brain structure, function, and AD pathologic features may be reduced among individuals with higher CR.[20–22] An important limitation of cross-sectional studies, however, is that they cannot test whether measures of CR alter future cognitive trajectories or the risk of cognitive impairment.

For this reason, prospective longitudinal studies that collect both AD biomarkers and cognitive and clinical data are essential for testing the extent to which CR is associated with reduced age-related cognitive decline or a reduced risk of cognitive impairment in the presence of AD pathologic features. The same factors that have been associated with CR (eg, educational and occupational attainment) may also minimize the accumulation of pathologic features, a concept known as brain maintenance,[23] which has been proposed as a complementary mechanism to CR. Thus, longitudinal studies addressing CR may also be relevant to the concept of brain maintenance.

LONGITUDINAL ALZHEIMER DISEASE BIOMARKER STUDIES OF COGNITIVE RESERVE AMONG INDIVIDUALS WITH NORMAL COGNITION WHEN FIRST EVALUATED

The number of prospective longitudinal studies that have investigated the relationship between measures of CR, AD biomarkers, and longitudinal cognitive or clinical outcomes among individuals who were cognitively normal at baseline is relatively limited (**Table 1**). These studies have examined the 3 major themes of (1) the association between baseline measures of CR and baseline AD biomarker levels in relation to the time to progress to cognitive impairment,[24–28] (2) the association between baseline measures of CR and baseline AD biomarker levels in relation to the rate of change in cognition,[13,29] and (3) the association between baseline measures of CR and the rate of change in AD biomarkers over time.[25,26,30,31]

Cognitive Reserve, Alzheimer Disease Biomarkers, and Risk of Cognitive Impairment

An important question that has been addressed by studies examining the first theme (the combined effects of CR and AD biomarkers on the risk of progression to cognitive impairment) is whether CR and AD biomarkers are independent predictors of risk or whether they interact to alter future risk of progression. The presence of such an interaction is very important because it would indicate that measures of CR modify the association between the biomarker and risk of progression, or that the protective effects of CR on the risk of progression differ for individuals with high versus low levels of the biomarker.

Two studies[24,26] addressed this question by testing whether the association between structural MRI measures of brain atrophy and the time to symptom onset of MCI is modified by CR, as quantified by a composite measure of CR (ie, a composite z-score composed of years of education, and measures of vocabulary and reading ability). Soldan and colleagues[26] (2015) found that the baseline volumes of 3 medial-temporal lobe structures (hippocampus, entorhinal cortex, and amygdala) and the rate of change in these structures over time, were associated with the time to progress from normal cognition to symptom onset of MCI, independently of the baseline CR composite score, which was associated with a reduced risk of progression (ie, delayed symptom onset). Only 1 structure, the left entorhinal cortex volume, interacted with CR, such that smaller baseline volumes were associated with faster

Table 1
Longitudinal studies of the association between cognitive reserve and Alzheimer biomarkers among individuals with normal cognition at baseline

Study	Outcome Variables	AD Biomarkers	CR Measures	Mean Clinical Follow-up Time in years (SD)	Number of Cognitively Normal Subjects at Baseline	Baseline CR-Biomarker Association	CR Associated with Delayed Clinical Progression or Better Cognitive Performance Accounting for Baseline Biomarker Levels	Longitudinal CR-Biomarker Association	Relationship Between Biomarker and Clinical or Cognitive Outcome Modified by CR
Soldan, et al,[13] 2017	Change in cognitive composite z-score	Composite z-score (CSF Aβ_{1-42}, p-tau, entorhinal cortex thickness, hippocampal volume, cortical thickness in AD-vulnerable regions)	Composite score (education, NART-IQ, WAIS-R vocabulary)	12.1 (4.2) max = 20	303 with clinical or cognitive data 170 with baseline biomarker data	No	Yes, better baseline cognitive performance and faster decline after MCI symptom onset	—	No
Pettigrew et al,[24] 2017	Time to onset of clinical symptom of MCI	Cortical thickness in AD vulnerable regions	Composite score (education, NART-IQ, WAIS-R vocabulary)	11.8 (3.6) max = 20	232 48 progressed	No	Yes Delayed clinical progression	—	Yes, for those who progressed 7 + years after baseline only
Soldan et al,[26] 2015	Time to onset of clinical symptom of MCI Change in AD biomarkers	Volumes of hippocampus, entorhinal cortex, amygdala Entorhinal cortex thickness	Composite score (education, NART-IQ, WAIS-R vocabulary)	11.1 (3.6), max = 18	245 57 progressed	No	Yes Delayed clinical progression	No	Yes, for left entorhinal cortex volume only

Study	Outcome	Biomarkers	CR measure	Follow-up (y)	N				
Vemuri et al,[29] 2015	Change in cognitive composite z-score	Cortical PiB-PET (dichotomous) White matter hyperintensity volume, brain infarcts on FLAIR-MRI (dichotomous)	Education or occupation score and self-reported midlife or late-life cognitive activity score	2.7	393	No	Yes, better baseline cognitive performance but no difference in slope	—	No
Soldan et al,[25] 2013	Time to onset of clinical symptom of MCI Change in AD biomarkers	CSF $A\beta_{1-42}$, t-tau, p-tau	Composite score (education, NART-IQ, WAIS-R vocabulary)	8.0 (3.4), max = 17	239, 53 progressed	No	Yes Delayed clinical progression	No	Yes, for CSF t-tau and p-tau
Suo et al,[31] 2012	Change in hippocampal volume	Hippocampal volume, whole-brain volume (VBM)	Lifetime Experiences Questionnaire (LEQ)	2–3, max = 3	151	Yes, midlife LEQ or occupational complexity and bilateral hippocampus, and left amygdala	—	Yes, high supervisory experiences associated with less hippocampal atrophy (N = 91)	—
Lo & Jagust,[30] 2013	Change AD biomarkers	CSF $A\beta_{1-42}$, t-tau, p-tau, FDG-PET metabolism in 5 AD-vulnerable regions, hippocampal volume	Education (tertiles), occupation (3 levels), NART errors (tertiles)	2–3, max = 3	229: 35 (CSF) 103 (FDG) 228 (HCV)	No	—	Yes, higher CR associated with less decline in CSF $A\beta_{1-42}$	—

(continued on next page)

Table 1
(continued)

Study	Outcome Variables	AD Biomarkers	CR Measures	Mean Clinical Follow-up Time in years (SD)	Number of Cognitively Normal Subjects at Baseline	Baseline CR-Biomarker Association	CR Associated with Delayed Clinical Progression or Better Cognitive Performance Accounting for Baseline Biomarker Levels	Longitudinal CR-Biomarker Association	Relationship Between Biomarker and Clinical or Cognitive Outcome Modified by CR
Roe et al,[27] 2011	Time to CDR ≥0.5 Change in CDR-SB, short Blessed Test, MMSE	CSF Aβ$_{1-42}$, t-tau, p-tau	Education	3.3 (2.0)	197 26 progressed	—	Yes, delayed clinical progression after accounting for Aβ$_{1-42}$, but not significant among those with low tau or p-tau Significant among those with high tau or p-tau	—	Yes, among those with high tau or p-tau and low education, WBV was associated with faster progression In low tau or p-tau group, neither education nor WBV associated with progression Similar results obtained for CDR-SB and Blessed Test, but not for MMSE
Roe et al,[28] 2011	Time to CDR ≥0.5	CSF Aβ$_{1-42}$, t-tau, p-tau	Education, occupational attainment (6 levels)	3.2 (1.6)	213 14 progressed	—	Yes Delayed clinical progression	—	—

Abbreviations: CDR, clinical dementia rating; CDR-SB, clinical dementia rating - sum of boxes score; CSF, cerebrospinal fluid; FDG, fluorodeoxyglucose; HVC, hippocampal volume; MCI, mild cognitive impairment; MMSE, Mini-Mental Status Exam; NART, National Adult Reading Test; VBM, voxel-based morphometry; WAIS-R, Wechsler Adult Intelligence Scale - revised; WBV, whole brain volume.

time to clinical symptom onset in individuals with low CR but not in individuals with high CR. Similar results were reported by Pettigrew and colleagues[24] (2017), who found that both CR and mean cortical thickness in AD-vulnerable regions were independently associated with risk of progression from normal cognition to MCI within 7 years of baseline. In contrast, there was an interaction between baseline CR score and cortical thickness for risk of progression more than 7 years from baseline, reflecting a stronger association between low cortical thickness and risk of symptom onset among individuals with lower CR. Additionally, they reported that the reduction in the risk of progression associated with higher CR was greater for progression after 7 years from baseline than for progression within 7 years, suggesting that the protective effect of CR decreases as AD pathologic features levels increase. Taken together, the results from these 2 studies suggest that MRI measures of atrophy in brain regions commonly affected by AD and measures of CR have relatively independent and additive effects on the risk of progression to MCI. However, these studies also provided some evidence for interactions between CR and atrophy in some brain regions, suggesting a stronger association between atrophy and risk among individuals with lower CR than higher CR.

Three other studies addressed this question by investigating the relationship between measures of CR and CSF measures of amyloid beta (Abeta), total tau (t-tau), and phosphorylated tau (p-tau) in relationship to the risk of progression to cognitive impairment.[25,27,28] For the findings regarding the relationship between CR and CSF Abeta, 2 of these studies reported that CR and CSF Abeta measures predicted time to progress from normal cognition to MCI but that there was no interaction between baseline levels of CSF Abeta and CR (as measured by years of education[27] or a composite score[25]). Similarly, the third study reported that fewer years of education and lower (ie, more abnormal) CSF Abeta levels were significantly associated with a faster time to onset of cognitive impairment; however, the interaction between the 2 measures was not examined.[28] Taken together, these findings suggest that the protective effects of CR on the risk of progression are equivalent across the observed range of CSF Abeta levels and that CR and Abeta have additive and independent effects on the risk of progression. This is noteworthy because CSF Abeta is widely accepted as a biomarker for amyloid plaques, a primary pathologic hallmark of AD.

The findings regarding the relationship between CR and CSF p-tau and t-tau suggest that there may be an interaction between CR and degree of neuronal injury, as measured by these biomarkers. Soldan and colleagues[25] (2013) found an interaction between the baseline CR composite score and both t-tau and p-tau in relationship to the time to onset of symptoms of MCI. Among participants with higher baseline levels of t-tau or p-tau, the degree to which CR modified the risk of symptom onset was less than that in participants with lower levels of t-tau and p-tau, though higher CR was still associated with a delay in symptom onset in both the low and high t-tau or p-tau groups. This suggests that, as levels of neuronal injury increase in the brain, the protective effects of CR decrease, consistent with the findings by Pettigrew and colleagues[24] (2017) using MRI measures of neuronal injury. This may occur because CR is unable to compensate for increasing levels of neuronal injury, or because the neural mechanisms that underlie CR break down with increasing levels of neuronal injury. The results by Soldan and colleagues[25] (2013) also indicated that CSF t-tau and p-tau levels were more strongly associated with the risk of progression among individuals with higher CR than those with lower CR. This was because individuals with lower CR were at significantly elevated risk of progressing (because of their low CR), even when t-tau or p-tau levels were low, and thus higher t-tau or p-tau levels were associated with less additional risk. By comparison, among those with higher

CR, whose overall risk of developing cognitive impairment is much lower, elevated tau or p-tau levels were more predictive of progression.

The findings by Roe and colleagues[27] (2011) were somewhat different. They reported a 3-way interaction between CR (as measured by years of education), t-tau or p-tau levels, and whole brain volume in relationship to the time to cognitive impairment. Among individuals with low t-tau or p-tau levels, there was no association between years of education and risk of progression; whereas, among individuals with high t-tau or p-tau levels, more education was associated with a delayed time to incident cognitive impairment, particularly among those with lower brain volumes. The 2-way interaction between t-tau or p-tau levels and education (collapsed across whole brain volume) was not reported. The absence of an association between education and risk of progression among those with low t-tau or p-tau levels may reflect the somewhat smaller sample size and smaller number of individuals who became symptomatic over the course of the study (which reduces statistical power) and the relatively short follow-up duration of 3 years (compared with 8 years in Soldan and colleagues,[25] 2013). Additionally, years of education alone tends to be less predictive of future cognitive impairment than composite CR measures that incorporate measures of literacy or vocabulary in addition to education.[24,32,33] The second study by Roe and colleagues[28] (2011) reported that both years of education and baseline t-tau or p-tau levels were predictive of incident cognitive impairment in the same model, although their possible interaction was not examined. Overall, the results of studies that have investigated the combined effects of CR and CSF AD biomarkers in relation to the risk of progression to MCI indicate that even after accounting for levels of these biomarkers at baseline, higher CR is associated with a reduced risk of symptom onset of MCI. Although the effects of Abeta and CR on the time to symptom onset seem to be independent of each another, there is some evidence that the protective effects of CR are modified by CSF t-tau and p-tau levels.

Cognitive Reserve, Alzheimer Disease Biomarker, and Rate of Cognitive Decline

Only 2 longitudinal studies have examined the previously mentioned second theme of the rate of change in neuropsychological measures of cognition in relationship to CR and AD biomarkers among individuals with normal cognition at baseline.[13,29] In both studies, cognitive performance was quantified with a composite z-score composed of measures from multiple cognitive domains. Vemuri and colleagues[29] (2015) operationalized CR in 2 ways, with 1 score reflecting educational and occupational attainment and the other indexing midlife and late-life cognitive leisure activities. The results showed that higher scores on the measure of educational and occupational attainment were associated with higher cognitive scores, independent of the amount of amyloid, as measured by PiB (Pittsburgh compound B)-PET imaging, as well as independent of cerebrovascular disease, as measured by white matter hyperintensities and brain infarcts on FLAIR (fluid attenuated inversion recovery)-MRI. Importantly, there was no interaction between the measures of CR and the MRI measures, suggesting similar rates of change in cognition over the follow-up period among those with higher and lower CR scores (mean follow-up 2.7 years). Consistent with these findings, Soldan and colleagues[13] (2017) also reported that, independent of AD biomarker levels, higher CR (as indexed by a composite score) was associated with better cognitive performance but did not alter the rates of cognitive change while individuals were asymptomatic (mean follow-up, 11 years). In this study, AD pathologic assessment was quantified by a composite score combining several major biomarker types (CSF Abeta and p-tau; as well as MRI measures of the hippocampus, entorhinal cortex, and AD-vulnerable cortical regions).

Due to the long follow-up period in this latter study, and that a substantial number of participants (66) had developed cognitive impairment on follow-up, Soldan and colleagues[13] (2017) also examined rates of change in cognition after the onset of symptoms of MCI. In line with theoretic predictions,[2] individuals with higher CR showed faster rates of cognitive decline than those with lower CR after they became symptomatic.[13] Additionally, the mean age of onset of symptoms of MCI was strongly associated with the baseline CR score: subjects with CR scores greater than the median had a mean age of symptom onset that was approximately 7 years later than for those with CR scores below the median of the group.[13] Notably, the subjects in this study were highly educated (mean of 17 years of education), so this study may underestimate the degree to which individual differences in CR may delay the symptomatic phase of AD. Taken together, the results from studies investigating the combined effects of CR and AD biomarkers on cognitive change and time to symptom onset suggest that, after accounting for baseline pathologic assessment levels, CR does not alter cognitive trajectories before symptom onset but does significantly delay the onset of symptoms by several years.

Cognitive Reserve and Rate of Change in Alzheimer Disease Biomarkers

Currently, there is weak evidence for the proposal that measures of CR are directly associated with the rate of change in AD biomarkers among individuals who were cognitively normal at baseline, the third previously mentioned theme. This is largely because the available data are limited by relatively short follow-up periods (2–4 years of longitudinal biomarker data, on average). Lo and Jagust[30] (2013) reported that, among a group of 35 cognitively normal individuals, higher scores on CR proxy variables (ie, measures of education, occupation, and reading or vocabulary) were associated with less longitudinal decline in CSF Abeta but not with change in MRI hippocampal volume or FDG (fluorodeoxyglucose) PET metabolism. Suo and colleagues[31] (2012) found that high self-reported supervisory experience in midlife (a measure assumed to reflect occupational complexity) was associated with less hippocampal atrophy over time in a sample of 91 older adults. However, self-reported general cognitive activities in early life, midlife, or late life did not modulate rates of brain atrophy. In 2 studies with larger samples (239 and 245), there was no relationship between a baseline CR composite and rates of change in CSF Abeta, t-tau, and p-tau,[25] or MRI measures of the hippocampus, amygdala, or entorhinal cortex.[26] Studies with large samples and more longitudinal biomarker data are needed to determine to what degree CR alters the trajectories of AD biomarkers and other aspects of brain health.

PATHWAYS LINKING COGNITIVE RESERVE TO COGNITIVE AND CLINICAL OUTCOMES

Despite the strong evidence that proxy measures of CR are associated with delayed clinical symptom onset, the mechanisms underlying these effects remain poorly understood. **Fig. 1** illustrates 4 possible pathways by which CR may alter longitudinal cognitive and clinical outcomes. First, CR may reduce the risk of MCI or dementia via mechanisms that are independent of the level of specific AD-related pathologic brain changes. For example, current evidence suggests that measures of CR and levels of brain amyloid independently predict the time to symptom onset.[25,27] Second, CR may interact with markers of pathologic features or brain health to influence future cognitive decline or risk of progression. For instance, smaller volumes or thickness in some AD vulnerable brain regions seem to be a stronger risk factor for developing cognitive impairment among individuals with low CR than for those with higher CR.[24,26] Also, the protective effects of CR on clinical outcomes seem to diminish as

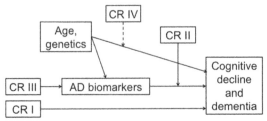

Fig. 1. Four possible pathways by which CR may influence rates of cognitive decline and risk of dementia in later life. CR refers to proxy measures such as educational or occupational attainment, as well as their neural implementations, which are not well understood. CR I is linked to outcomes in a way that is unrelated to biomarker levels. CR II moderates the relationship between biomarkers and outcomes. CR III has a direct effect on biomarker levels (ie, onset or rate of accumulation). CR IV modifies the relationship between age or genetics and outcomes. Dashed line indicates that, although illustrated as a moderation effect, it could be a mediation effect or the relationship may depend on a specific demographic factor, gene, or so forth.

levels of neuronal injury increase,[25] suggesting that the neural mechanisms of CR become overwhelmed by disease. A third pathway by which CR may influence future cognitive and clinical outcomes is by delaying the onset of age-related or AD-related brain changes, or reducing the rate of AD pathologic feature accumulation. Although current evidence for this pathway is limited, future studies with longer follow-up periods will be able to investigate this pathway. For example, recent evidence suggests that midlife vascular risk factors, including obesity, high cholesterol, hypertension, and smoking, are associated with late-life amyloid accumulation.[34] To the extent that these midlife vascular risk factors are associated with CR proxy measures, such as educational or occupational attainment,[35–37] CR may influence the accumulation of AD pathologic features indirectly via health-related behaviors in early life and midlife. A fourth pathway that has been proposed is that CR alters the association between genetic factors or aging on clinical and cognitive outcomes. Older age is the greatest risk factor for AD and both amyloid and tau pathologic features increase with age. Preliminary evidence from cross-sectional studies suggests that the association between age and AD pathologic feature levels[20] or age-related structural brain changes[21,22] may be attenuated among individuals with higher CR.

An important limitation of current longitudinal studies is that they have not yet fully explored the neural mechanisms of CR. Evidence from cross-sectional suggests that CR may be implemented in the brain in the form of greater neural efficiency and speed,[38–40] neural capacity, neural compensation,[39,41] and greater functional connectivity.[42] Longitudinal studies will be necessary to test whether these putative mechanisms of CR are associated with better clinical outcomes, in the same way as proxy measures of CR. If so, it might be possible to devise interventions that specifically target these neural mechanisms, thereby increasing reserve and resilience of the brain.

COGNITIVE RESERVE AND PUBLIC HEALTH: PRACTICAL IMPLICATIONS

The study of CR and its neural implementation has important implications for public health. To the extent that higher CR protects against the clinical manifestations of AD by delaying the onset of the symptomatic phase of the disease, it provides an important mechanism for preserving cognitive function in old age, even while the level of brain pathologic features is rising. Current evidence suggests that higher CR is associated with an approximately 50% reduction in the relative risk of symptom onset of MCI[24–26,33] and may delay the onset of symptoms by several years.[13] As such, CR provides far greater potential benefits to individuals than any drug that is currently on the market for treating the symptoms of MCI or dementia. Moreover, by delaying the onset of the symptomatic phase of AD, CR allows older individuals to maximize daily functioning and minimize reliance on caregivers. Caring for someone with dementia is associated with enormous stress, financial strain, and negative health outcomes. Therefore, the goal of any intervention for AD should be to prolong the time that older adults are able to live independently and be active and engaged members of their family and community. Moreover, the current findings regarding CR suggest that health policies aimed at improving educational and occupational opportunities for individuals may have far-reaching consequences for future rates of cognitive decline and dementia.

REFERENCES

1. Stern Y, Alexander GE, Prohovnik I, et al. Inverse relationship between education and parietotemporal perfusion deficit in Alzheimer's disease. Ann Neurol 1992; 32(3):371–5.
2. Stern Y. Cognitive reserve. Neuropsychologia 2009;47(10):2015–28.
3. Perneczky R, Drzezga A, Boecker H, et al. Activities of daily living, cerebral glucose metabolism, and cognitive reserve in Lewy body and Parkinson's disease. Dement Geriatr Cogn Disord 2008;26(5):475–81.
4. Sumowski JF, Rocca MA, Leavitt VM, et al. Brain reserve and cognitive reserve protect against cognitive decline over 4.5 years in MS. Neurology 2014;82(20): 1776–83.
5. Mathias JL, Wheaton P. Contribution of brain or biological reserve and cognitive or neural reserve to outcome after TBI: a meta-analysis (prior to 2015). Neurosci Biobehav Rev 2015;55:573–93.
6. Barulli D, Stern Y. Efficiency, capacity, compensation, maintenance, plasticity: emerging concepts in cognitive reserve. Trends Cogn Sci 2013;17(10):502–9.
7. Sperling RA, Aisen PS, Beckett LA, et al. Toward defining the preclinical stages of Alzheimer's disease: recommendations from the National Institute on Aging-Alzheimer's Association workgroups on diagnostic guidelines for Alzheimer's disease. Alzheimers Dement 2011;7(3):280–92.
8. Brookmeyer R, Gray S, Kawas C. Projections of Alzheimer's disease in the United States and the public health impact of delaying disease onset. Am J Public Health 1998;88(9):1337–42.
9. Stern Y, Gurland B, Tatemichi TK, et al. Influence of education and occupation on the incidence of Alzheimer's disease. JAMA 1994;271(13):1004–10.
10. Andel R, Crowe M, Pedersen NL, et al. Complexity of work and risk of Alzheimer's disease: a population-based study of Swedish twins. J Gerontol B Psychol Sci Soc Sci 2005;60(5):P251–8.
11. Wilson RS, Mendes De Leon CF, Barnes LL, et al. Participation in cognitively stimulating activities and risk of incident Alzheimer disease. JAMA 2002;287(6): 742–8.
12. Zahodne LB, Glymour MM, Sparks C, et al. Education does not slow cognitive decline with aging: 12-year evidence from the Victoria longitudinal study. J Int Neuropsychol Soc 2011;17(6):1039–46.

13. Soldan A, Pettigrew C, Cai Q, et al. Cognitive reserve and long-term change in cognition in aging and preclinical Alzheimer's disease. Neurobiol Aging 2017; 60:164–72.

14. Liu Y, Julkunen V, Paajanen T, et al. Education increases reserve against Alzheimer's disease–evidence from structural MRI analysis. Neuroradiology 2012; 54(9):929–38.

15. Querbes O, Aubry F, Pariente J, et al. Early diagnosis of Alzheimer's disease using cortical thickness: impact of cognitive reserve. Brain 2009;132(Pt 8):2036–47.

16. Sole-Padulles C, Bartres-Faz D, Junque C, et al. Brain structure and function related to cognitive reserve variables in normal aging, mild cognitive impairment and Alzheimer's disease. Neurobiol Aging 2009;30(7):1114–24.

17. Rentz DM, Mormino EC, Papp KV, et al. Cognitive resilience in clinical and preclinical Alzheimer's disease: the Association of Amyloid and Tau Burden on cognitive performance. Brain Imaging Behav 2017;11(2):383–90.

18. Roe CM, Mintun MA, D'Angelo G, et al. Alzheimer disease and cognitive reserve: variation of education effect with carbon 11-labeled Pittsburgh Compound B uptake. Arch Neurol 2008;65(11):1467–71.

19. Dumurgier J, Paquet C, Benisty S, et al. Inverse association between CSF Abeta 42 levels and years of education in mild form of Alzheimer's disease: the cognitive reserve theory. Neurobiol Dis 2010;40(2):456–9.

20. Almeida RP, Schultz SA, Austin BP, et al. Effect of cognitive reserve on age-related changes in cerebrospinal fluid biomarkers of Alzheimer Disease. JAMA Neurol 2015;72(6):699–706.

21. Steffener J, Habeck C, O'Shea D, et al. Differences between chronological and brain age are related to education and self-reported physical activity. Neurobiol Aging 2016;40:138–44.

22. Habeck C, Razlighi Q, Gazes Y, et al. Cognitive reserve and brain maintenance: orthogonal concepts in theory and practice. Cereb Cortex 2016;27(8):3962–9.

23. Nyberg L, Lovden M, Riklund K, et al. Memory aging and brain maintenance. Trends Cogn Sci 2012;16(5):292–305.

24. Pettigrew C, Soldan A, Zhu Y, et al. Cognitive reserve and cortical thickness in preclinical Alzheimer's disease. Brain Imaging Behav 2017;11(2):357–67.

25. Soldan A, Pettigrew C, Li S, et al. Relationship of cognitive reserve and cerebrospinal fluid biomarkers to the emergence of clinical symptoms in preclinical Alzheimer's disease. Neurobiol Aging 2013;34(12):2827–34.

26. Soldan A, Pettigrew C, Lu Y, et al. Relationship of medial temporal lobe atrophy, APOE genotype, and cognitive reserve in preclinical Alzheimer's disease. Hum Brain Mapp 2015;36(7):2826–41.

27. Roe CM, Fagan AM, Grant EA, et al. Cerebrospinal fluid biomarkers, education, brain volume, and future cognition. Arch Neurol 2011;68(9):1145–51.

28. Roe CM, Fagan AM, Williams MM, et al. Improving CSF biomarker accuracy in predicting prevalent and incident Alzheimer disease. Neurology 2011;76(6): 501–10.

29. Vemuri P, Lesnick TG, Przybelski SA, et al. Vascular and amyloid pathologies are independent predictors of cognitive decline in normal elderly. Brain 2015;138(Pt 3):761–71.

30. Lo RY, Jagust WJ. Effect of cognitive reserve markers on Alzheimer pathologic progression. Alzheimer Dis Assoc Disord 2013;27(4):343–50.

31. Suo C, Leon I, Brodaty H, et al. Supervisory experience at work is linked to low rate of hippocampal atrophy in late life. Neuroimage 2012;63(3):1542–51.

32. Manly JJ, Schupf N, Tang MX, et al. Cognitive decline and literacy among ethnically diverse elders. J Geriatr Psychiatry Neurol 2005;18(4):213–7.

33. Pettigrew C, Soldan A, Li S, et al. Relationship of cognitive reserve and APOE status to the emergence of clinical symptoms in preclinical Alzheimer's disease. Cogn Neurosci 2013;4(3–4):136–42.

34. Gottesman RF, Schneider AL, Zhou Y, et al. Association between midlife vascular risk factors and estimated brain amyloid deposition. JAMA 2017;317(14): 1443–50.

35. Smith JP. The impact of socioeconomic status on health over the life-course. J Hum Resour 2007;42(4):739–64.

36. Devaux M, Sassi F, Church J, et al. Exploring the relationship between education and obesity. OECD Economic Studies 2011;1:1–40.

37. Non AL, Gravlee CC, Mulligan CJ. Education, genetic ancestry, and blood pressure in African Americans and Whites. Am J Public Health 2012;102(8):1559–65.

38. Speer ME, Soldan A. Cognitive reserve modulates ERPs associated with verbal working memory in healthy younger and older adults. Neurobiol Aging 2015; 36(3):1424–34.

39. Steffener J, Reuben A, Rakitin BC, et al. Supporting performance in the face of age-related neural changes: testing mechanistic roles of cognitive reserve. Brain Imaging Behav 2011;5(3):212–21.

40. Habeck C, Hilton HJ, Zarahn E, et al. Relation of cognitive reserve and task performance to expression of regional covariance networks in an event-related fMRI study of nonverbal memory. Neuroimage 2003;20(3):1723–33.

41. Stern Y, Zarahn E, Habeck C, et al. A common neural network for cognitive reserve in verbal and object working memory in young but not old. Cereb Cortex 2008;18(4):959–67.

42. Arenaza-Urquijo EM, Landeau B, La Joie R, et al. Relationships between years of education and gray matter volume, metabolism and functional connectivity in healthy elders. Neuroimage 2013;83:450–7.

Electroconvulsive Therapy in Geriatric Psychiatry

A Selective Review

Justin P. Meyer, MD[a],*, Samantha K. Swetter, MD[a],
Charles H. Kellner, MD[b]

KEYWORDS

- Electroconvulsive therapy • ECT • Geriatric • Depression • Dementia • Cognition
- Parkinson's

KEY POINTS

- Electroconvulsive therapy (ECT) is a safe and effective treatment of geriatric patients with severe depressive illness, mania, schizophrenia, and some neuropsychiatric conditions.
- The cognitive effects of ECT are largely transient, even in elderly patients with premorbid impairment.
- ECT does not worsen the course of dementia, and is indicated for comorbid depression and agitation in dementia.
- Medical comorbidities in the older adult population may increase risk and must be considered before ECT, but do not preclude its use.

INTRODUCTION

Electroconvulsive therapy (ECT) remains an important treatment of geriatric patients with severe depressive illness and a limited number of other severe psychiatric conditions. As the United States population continues to age, the burden of psychiatric illness in this age group will continue to increase. Since its introduction, ECT has been one of the most effective treatments for psychiatric illness across demographics.[1] Numerous studies have indicated that ECT may be more effective in the elderly than in other age groups.[2–4] Therefore, ECT must be a treatment consideration in the elderly, particularly in instances of medication resistance or intolerance. In

Disclosure: C.H. Kellner has received grant support from the NIMH; receives honoraria from Cambridge University Press; and receives fees from Psychiatric Times, UpToDate, and the Northwell Health System. J.P. Meyer and S.K. Swetter have nothing to disclose.
a Department of Psychiatry, Icahn School of Medicine at Mount Sinai, 1 Gustave Levy Place, Box 1230, New York, NY 10029, USA; b Department of Electroconvulsive Therapy (ECT), New York Community Hospital, 2525 Kings Highway, Brooklyn, NY 11229, USA
* Corresponding author.
E-mail address: Justin.meyer@mssm.edu

addition, ECT serves a vital role in treating urgent illness requiring expedient recovery, such as catatonia, or in patients with severe suicidal ideation or intent. Despite concerns regarding increasing medical comorbidities in the geriatric population, ECT remains a fairly safe treatment option with few medical contraindications.[5] The evidence base supports ECT's use as an effective treatment in a variety of neuropsychiatric conditions in the elderly, including depression, mania, psychosis, catatonia, and Parkinson's disease (PD).

Despite ECT's efficacy, concerns regarding its side effect burden may reduce its appeal. Many clinicians remain concerned about the cognitive effects of ECT, particularly retrograde amnesia, in an aging population whose memory function may be compromised at baseline. Recent studies have examined the relationship of ECT to preexisting memory impairment and, contrary to prior assumptions, indicate that ECT may not significantly worsen these difficulties.[4,6–9]

There has been considerable progress elucidating ECT's mechanism of action.[10–12] ECT uses an electrical stimulus to induce depolarization of cerebral neurons, causing a seizure in an anesthetized patient. Inducing a generalized seizure via ECT also has acute systemic effects, which must be managed in geriatric patients, who may have numerous medical comorbidities. Broadly, sympathetic tone increases during seizure development, whereas vagal tone increases at the time of the stimulus and at seizure termination. This autonomic shift may strain the cardiovascular system.[13–15] Given the potential cardiovascular stress and the use of general anesthesia, specific attention must be paid to these concerns when evaluating geriatric patients for ECT.

METHODS

The authors searched the PubMed database for "electroconvulsive therapy elderly," "electroconvulsive therapy geriatric," "ECT elderly," and "ECT geriatric" with the addition of the terms reviewed later ("unipolar," "bipolar," "mania," "major depressive disorder," "catatonia," "schizophrenia," "psychosis," and "dementia"). If no data specific to the geriatric population were available, citations referring to mixed-age populations were used, and so noted in the article. Citations with content not relevant to this article were excluded.

PHYSIOLOGY OF ELECTROCONVULSIVE THERAPY

ECT uses an electrical stimulus to induce a seizure in an anesthetized patient. This seizure results in beneficial and adverse physiologic changes in the brain and other organs. Although the physiology of ECT in the elderly remains largely the same as in the general population, there are a few notable differences. First, age increases the seizure threshold (ST). The increased ST in the elderly may be caused by several factors, including decreased excitability of the brain and increased skull thickness.[16,17] Regardless of the precise cause, an increased ST requires higher stimulus intensity to elicit an adequate seizure. Older adults also tend to have shorter seizure duration, shorter slow-wave-phase duration, and overall weaker seizure strength, based on electroencephalogram morphology with less clear onset and offset of seizure.[16,17]

Electrode Placement

Three electrode placements have become standard in contemporary ECT practice: bilateral (BL), also referred to as bitemporal, right unilateral (RUL), and bifrontal. Other placements have been used clinically and experimentally but none has entered common clinical practice.[18] Left unilateral electrode placement may be considered in those rare cases of left-handed patients with right hemisphere language dominance.[19]

Left anterior, right temporal placement has also been promoted by some clinicians as a clinically viable alternative.[20] The clinical efficacy and adverse effect profile of ECT is affected by electrode placement. In general, BL ECT is associated with higher remission rates, greater speed of response/remission, and greater cognitive effects. In contrast, RUL, although it may approach the efficacy of BL, is typically associated with fewer cognitive effects.[18] Theoretically, this difference is presumed to be caused by different current paths/density in the brain, with RUL sparing the language centers in the dominant (left) hemisphere.[21]

The choice between RUL and BL remains particularly complex in the elderly.[22] However, there are limited data in the elderly population comparing RUL with BL ECT. Fraser and Glass[23] randomized 29 elderly depressed patients to receive twice-weekly RUL or BL ECT. Similar to the general population, they found no difference in efficacy or memory performance following the treatment course. Many recent studies have found RUL ECT to be an effective treatment in these patients.[4] The choice between RUL and BL ECT in the elderly hinges on numerous factors, including severity of symptoms, medical comorbidities, and the patient's ongoing response to treatment.[14] Therefore, the decision to treat with unilateral or bilateral placements should be made on an individual basis through a thorough discussion of the risks and benefits with the patients and their families.[22]

Stimulus Dosing/Stimulus Parameters

Electrical stimulus dosing in ECT is analogous to medication dosing in pharmacotherapy. Although there is no perfect summary unit to fully describe the electrical stimulus package, the field has adopted charge to compare electrical doses. The stimulus dosing strategy is in part determined by the electrode placement, with RUL ECT likely requiring at least 2.5 times the ST stimulus (and typically up to 6–8 times ST) for maximal antidepressant efficacy. BL ECT likely requires at least 1.5 times ST.[17] In cases of poor clinical response, the stimulus may be increased.[24] Because the elderly tend to have an increased ST, they may require a higher stimulus, which is associated with increased cognitive difficulties following treatment.[24] In addition, the individual components of the stimulus package (current, frequency, pulse width, and train duration) can influence both efficacy and adverse effects. In clinical practice, the use of ultrabrief pulse (UBP) stimuli (defined as <0.5 milliseconds), particularly with RUL electrode placement, has become common. Given these data, many clinicians' approach is to begin with RUL, either ultrabrief or brief pulse, but to switch to BL if RUL is ineffective or response is slow.[22] If intolerable cognitive side effects do develop with BL, the patient may be switched back to RUL, or the treatment discontinued.[22]

INDICATIONS
Unipolar and Bipolar Depression

ECT is the most common and effective modality for treatment-resistant depression, in the context of either unipolar or bipolar depressive episodes. In addition, it may be used as a first-line treatment in patients who present with urgent or life-threatening depressive illness, when speed of response is crucial. Studies of ECT in the elderly indicate response rates greater than 63% (**Table 1**). Spaans and colleagues[25] found that geriatric depressed patients receiving ECT achieved remission faster and had a significantly higher remission rate: 63.8%, compared with 33.3% for medication. Furthermore, no trial has reported antidepressant medications to be more effective than ECT. The Prolonging Remission in Depressed Elderly (PRIDE) study provides some of the newest and most comprehensive evidence of ECT's efficacy. The first

Table 1
A selective review of electroconvulsive therapy in geriatric depression

Author, Year	Study Design	Sample Size	Age (y)	Methods	Primary Outcome	Results
Coffey et al,[81] 1989	Prospective	51	60–90 (mean 71.3)	ECT 3 times weekly, mixed placement, 9 mean ECT treatments	Response on MADRS score	82% full therapeutic response
Rubin et al,[82] 1991	Retrospective	101	Mean 76.0	46% received ECT ± antidepressant therapy	BDI score	Compared with drug therapy, ECT had significantly lower final BDI scores, a greater reduction in BDI scores
Mulsant et al,[83] 1991	Prospective	42	60–89 (mean 73.5)	ECT 3 times weekly; unilateral (n = 29), bilateral (n = 3), both (n = 10), 8.3 mean ECT treatments, (range 4–13)	BPRS score	38 patients with decreased BPRS score
Kellner et al,[84] 1992	RCT	15	53–87 (mean 69.9)	Randomized to weekly or 3 times weekly bilateral ECT for 3 wk	Blinded HAM-D score	Mean HAM-D decreased 27–12 in 3 times/wk ECT and 29–20 in weekly ECT
Wilkinson et al,[85] 1993	Prospective	43 patients >65 y	>65	ECT twice weekly; mostly bilateral; 7.9 mean treatments	≥50% reduction in MADRS score	73% ≥65 y old, 54% <65 y
Tomac et al,[86] 1997	Retrospective	34 patients >85 y	Mean 81	ECT 3 times weekly; 7 mean ECT treatments; mostly unilateral	GAF score, HRSD score, BPRS score	Significant GAF increase by mean 8.2 points (n = 30), significant HAM-D decrease by mean 5.7 points (n = 16), significant BPRS decrease by mean 47.2 points (n = 18)
Tew et al,[87] 1999	Prospective	268 women	63 patients aged 60–74; 72 patients aged ≥75	ECT 3 times weekly; unilateral (n = 136), bilateral (n = 22), both (n = 87)	HAM-D score ≤10 3 d post-ECT	≥75 y, 67%; aged 60–74 y, 73%; <60 y, 54%

Study	Design	N	Age	Description	CGI score	Outcome
Damm et al,[88] 2010	Retrospective	114 patients >60 y	Mixed adults	Chart review of effect of age on outcome		Considerable improvement in all age groups
Rhebergen et al,[2] 2015	Prospective	120	Mixed adults	Twice-weekly RUL ECT for depression	HAM-D score rate of change at 6-wk follow-up	Rapid remission group's mean age was 65.3 y compared with 57.6 y for the moderate response group and 51.5 y for the nonremitting group
Spaans et al,[25] 2015	Secondary Analysis of data from Two RCTs	47 ECT, 81 pharmacotherapy	Mean 74.0 for ECT, mean 72.2 for pharmacotherapy	6-wk ECT vs 12-wk pharmacotherapy for treatment of unipolar depression	Remission on MADRS	ECT patients remitted a mean of 3.07 wk faster (P = .008) with a remission rate of 63.8% compared with 33.3%
Bjolseth et al,[89] 2016	Prospective	57	60–85	Mixed electrode placement for unipolar and bipolar major depressive episodes	HAM-D score from baseline to after ECT treatment	Mean decrease in HAM-D score was 14.7 points
Kellner et al,[4] 2016	Prospective	240	>60	RUL UBP ECT combined with venlafaxine	Remission on HAM-D	61.7% remission rate
Kellner et al,[8] 2016	RCT	120	>60	Venlafaxine + lithium ± continuation ECT for remitters from phase 1	HAM-D score at 24 wk	Statistically significant mean end treatment score of 5.5 in medication + ECT group compared with 9.4 in medication group
Rosen et al,[3] 2016	Retrospective	482	Mixed adults	Chart review of rehospitalization rates of patients ≥65 y old compared with those <65 y old	Rehospitalization within last 5 y	Geriatric group with lower rehospitalization rates (6.2%) compared with nongeriatric patients (22%), P<.0001

Abbreviations: BDI, Beck Depression Inventory; BPRS, Brief Psychiatric Rating Scale; CGI, Clinical Global Impression; GAF, Global Assessment of Functioning; HAM-D, Hamilton Depression Rating Scale; HSRD, Hamilton Rating Scale for Depression; MADRS, Montgomery-Åsberg Depression Rating Scale; RCT, randomized controlled trial.

phase of the study included 240 patients more than 60 years of age who received UBP RUL ECT in combination with venlafaxine. Sixty-two percent of patients remitted and 70% responded. The mean number of treatments to achieve remission was 7.3.[4] Data for the general population indicate that ECT is as effective for bipolar depression as it is in a major depressive episode; this response is likely similar for the geriatric population.[1]

Older age has repeatedly been shown to positively predict speed and response to ECT.[26] The PRIDE study confirmed this finding, noting that patients more than 70 years old were 1.89 times more likely to respond than those 60 to 69 years old, and a larger portion of those greater than 70 years old remitted (69.7%) compared with those who were 60 to 69 years old (55.0%).[4] Others also suggest that older age is associated with more rapid and complete remission.[2,3] The reason for the improved response in the elderly is unclear but is likely multifactorial, including lower rates of comorbid personality disorder, higher rates of medication intolerance, and perhaps earlier referral to ECT.[26]

The PRIDE study also examined other predictors of response. A change in the Hamilton Depression Rating Scale (HAM-D) score following the first ECT predicted outcome in a dose response fashion: each 1-point increment change on the HAM-D correlated with a 5% increased odds of remission at the end of treatment.[4] In addition, individuals with Beck Scale of Suicidal Ideation scores of 0 at baseline were twice (odds ratio, 2.0) as likely to remit as those with scores greater than 0.[4]

Numerous studies in the mixed adult population have found other predictors of ECT response that likely also apply to the older population. Adults with psychotic depression respond better to ECT.[26] In contrast, adults with increased depressive episode length and chronicity of illness have a less robust response to ECT.[26] Recently, Oudega and colleagues[27–29] suggested that severe medial temporal lobe atrophy seen on MRI may be inversely correlated to ECT response, whereas white matter disease in other regions may not be associated with this change. However, these and other imaging studies are small, with unclear clinical significance, and await replication.[30,31]

Mania

ECT is an effective treatment of mania. Although pharmacotherapy remains the first-line treatment of mania, ECT should be considered in urgent situations. There are limited data regarding ECT's use in the elderly with mania. In the general population, ECT seems to be more effective than conservative management for mania, with a reduction in length of stay and symptoms.[32] In mixed-age adult populations, studies have also found ECT to be superior to drug therapy (up to 80% effective), particularly if the patient is treatment refractory to medication.[33,34] Other data indicate that ECT may be most effective for agitated mania or mixed states, which tend to occur in chronic illness and are more often the case in the elderly.[35]

Catatonia

Catatonia, characterized by disturbed motor activity (eg, cataplexy, waxy flexibility, mutism), previously considered a subtype of schizophrenia, is now known to occur most commonly in the context of serious mood disorder or medical illness, and is more common in the elderly.[36,37] Benzodiazepines typically represent the first-line treatment of catatonia and are effective 60% to 70% of the time.[36] However, patients may become tolerant, making this treatment less effective. ECT should also be considered as a first-line intervention for catatonia in cases of severe illness, such as malignant catatonia, neuroleptic malignant syndrome, delirious mania, or severe catatonic excitement.[37]

ECT remains a definitive treatment of catatonia in the general population, with responses ranging from 80% to 100% in numerous case series, regardless of comorbidity or underlying diagnosis.[37–39] However, there are limited data explicitly examining geriatric patients with catatonia treated with ECT, but a case series by Suzuki and colleagues[40] suggests that it is as effective in the elderly as in the general population. In mixed adult populations, it seems catatonia responds best to ECT when associated with a mood disorder rather than a psychotic disorder.[41]

Psychotic Spectrum Illness

Adults with treatment-refractory psychotic spectrum illness, including schizophrenia, also respond well to ECT. However, there are no randomized controlled data examining the elderly with psychotic spectrum disorders. Prospective trials indicate that bilateral ECT is a safe and effective treatment in older adults with schizophrenia.[42] In the general adult population, data robustly support the use of ECT in treatment-refractory schizophrenia. Several studies have compared ECT in combination with antipsychotic medication with sham ECT with antipsychotic medication; all found ECT superior to sham. ECT plus medication reduced symptoms of psychosis and maintained this gain, resulting in fewer relapses and less time hospitalized.[43] More recently, studies show antipsychotics are safe and synergistic with ECT.[43–46]

Across demographics, the best evidence for the use of ECT in schizophrenia exists in cases with comorbid catatonia, aggression, acute onset of illness, short duration, or significant suicidality when a rapid response is required.[43] ECT also has a greater effect on the positive rather than negative symptoms of schizophrenia.

Neurologic Illnesses (Major Neurocognitive Disorder with Comorbid Depression, Parkinson's Disease, Poststroke Depression, Agitation in Dementia and Delirium)

ECT has a rich tradition of use in neurologic illnesses, including major neurocognitive disorder or dementia with comorbid depression, Parkinson's disease (PD), movement disorders, poststroke depression, and agitation in dementia and delirium.

Up to 50% of patients with dementia also have depressive symptoms; for many, this represents their first affective episode.[1,47] ECT remains efficacious for these depressive symptoms and evidence suggests that although ECT may be associated with transient cognitive effects, it does not hasten the course of the dementia.[48,49] The diagnosis of depression in dementia is complicated by the fact that presentations may be atypical and patients may be unable to express subjective feelings of depression.[1] The choice of electrode placement for the treatment of depression in dementia is like that for other indications. If there are concerns about transient worsening of cognition, RUL can be used; however, BL should be considered if the patient is urgently or very medically ill.[14]

As with dementia, patients with PD commonly have comorbid depression.[47] Numerous case reports and series indicate that ECT is a safe and effective treatment of both the motor and depressive symptoms in PD.[50,51] Because of this, ECT is a particularly attractive treatment option for these patients. The mechanism of ECT's effects in PD is likely related to dopaminergic enhancement.[52–55] RUL is preferred in patients with PD because it is less likely to induce delirium.[14] For this reason, dopaminergic medications should also be decreased during a course of ECT. Because the beneficial effect of ECT on motor symptoms is transient, continuation and maintenance ECT should be considered in appropriately selected patients with PD.[50] ECT may also aid in the treatment of the motor, depressive, and psychotic symptoms of dementia with Lewy bodies.[56] Other motor disorders, including Tourette, tardive dyskinesia, and tardive dystonia, have been reported to be improved with ECT.[57,58]

ECT also has established efficacy for depression following stroke. Poststroke depression occurs in one-third of patients in the first 2 years following a stroke. A substantial literature shows that ECT can safely and effectively treat these patients.[59,60]

An emerging literature suggests that ECT is also an effective and well-tolerated treatment of agitation in dementia when other treatment modalities have failed.[61–64] If ECT is effective in treating agitation in dementia, then continuation/maintenance ECT may be needed to sustain this benefit.[62] Because many of these patients are unable to provide fully informed consent, a careful process to obtain substituted consent is crucial.

For delirium of various causes, ECT can provide important symptomatic relief regardless of the underlying cause. This usage of ECT has been particularly popular in Europe and should occur in parallel with a medical work-up to diagnose/treat the medical cause of the delirium.[63,64]

ACUTE, CONTINUATION, AND MAINTENANCE ELECTROCONVULSIVE THERAPY

An acute course of ECT, administered 2 or 3 times per week, is designed to treat an episode of mood disorder or other acute symptom presentations; continuation/maintenance ECT is the administration of single ECT sessions (usually on an outpatient basis) at intervals to prevent relapse or recurrence of symptoms. The average acute course of ECT consists of 3 treatments a week for a total of 6 to 12 treatments.[65] However, this course may vary depending on the patient's treatment response and side effects. ECT should be stopped when the patient has either remitted or improvement has plateaued.[65]

Following the acute course, the patient may be offered continuation ECT, in combination with pharmacotherapy and/or psychotherapy, depending on the patient's history and preferences. Because of the high rate of relapse (up to 50%) in the months following a course of ECT, current evidence suggests that acute ECT should be tapered before discontinuation.[26,66] Therefore, for selected patients, ECT may be reduced in frequency but continued in the 6 months following the acute course. The precise duration and frequency of continuation, like acute phase ECT, is determined by the individual's symptoms and history. If the patient does not experience recurrence of symptoms, then ECT may be further spaced out, but if the patient experiences worsening illness then frequency may be increased.[66]

Similar to acute ECT, continuation ECT seems to be safe and effective in the older adult population.[67] The second phase of the PRIDE trial examined a novel schedule of continuation ECT in elderly depressed patients following an acute course of UBP RUL ECT. Remitted individuals were randomized to receive either venlafaxine plus lithium or continuation ECT in combination with those medications. The continuation ECT group received 4 continuation ECT treatments in the first month following remission, with a provision to receive additional rescue ECT for symptom recurrence in the following 5 months. Individuals who received ECT in combination with medication had significantly fewer depressive symptoms as measured by the HAM-D, and more were rated not ill at all on the Clinical Global Impressions severity scale compared with those receiving medication alone.[8]

Following the 6-month continuation phase, patients may be considered for maintenance ECT. Maintenance treatments should be kept at the minimum frequency required to sustain remission.[26] The decision to pursue maintenance ECT is based on risk factors for relapse. The number of previous episodes of illness, medication resistance, and psychotic depression all increase the probability of relapse.[26] Similarly, the patient's illness severity or symptom profile, such as suicidality, may suggest a need for maintenance ECT. Maintenance ECT in affectively ill elderly patients reduces relapses, leading to fewer rehospitalizations.[68] Similarly, maintenance ECT effectively reduces readmission and length of hospitalization in the elderly with psychotic spectrum illness (eg, schizophrenia or severe affective illness).[69] Taken together, continuation and maintenance ECT is a safe and effective treatment to prevent relapse of chronic mental illness in the elderly.

ADVERSE EFFECTS

ECT is a generally safe and well-tolerated treatment. The most common side effects are headache, muscle ache, and nausea.[44,70] Like any procedure under general anesthesia, ECT carries the risk of more serious adverse events, including prolonged seizure and death. Mortality with ECT is extremely rare, occurring with an incidence of 2.1 in 100,000 treatments or about 1 in 10,000 patients.[5,44] Cardiac dysfunction (eg, myocardial infarction, congestive heart failure, valvular disease), cerebral abnormalities (eg, cerebrovascular malformation, lesions with increased intracranial pressure, recent stroke/hemorrhage), and respiratory disease (eg, chronic obstructive pulmonary disease, asthma, pneumonia, or an American Society of Anesthesiologists level 4 or 5 classification) increase mortality risk. Although age does not seem to be an independent risk factor for mortality caused by ECT, older adults are at increased risk because of the increased prevalence of medical comorbidities.[71]

TOLERABILITY
Cognition

Cognitive impairment remains ECT's most concerning side effect to practitioners and patients. The cognitive effects of ECT may include an acute confusional state, as well as anterograde and retrograde amnesia.

The acute confusional state occurs immediately following the treatment and is likely caused by both the seizure and anesthesia. It typically lasts no longer than 1 hour.[26] Age, gray and white matter disease, and dementia, particularly PD, may prolong this confusion.[14]

Anterograde amnesia, or the inability to retain new memories, typically resolves within 1 to 3 weeks after a course of ECT.[14,26] Retrograde amnesia, or the forgetting of the events before the ECT, also tends to resolve, with the patient recovering many of these memories over this time frame. Risk factors for worsened anterograde and retrograde amnesia during treatment include increased age, brain disease, limited cognitive reserve, and prolonged acute confusional state. Treatment parameters are also associated with worsened anterograde and retrograde amnesia; these include increased stimulus intensity and treatment frequency, and bilateral electrode placement.[14,26]

Studies suggest that although ECT affects cognition during the acute treatment period, these effects resolve without long-term changes in cognition, even in the elderly.[4,6–9] A small subset of patients report a more profound subjective retrograde amnestic syndrome with unclear cause or predictive factors.[14,72]

Cardiovascular

The most serious adverse events associated with ECT in the elderly population involve the cardiovascular system. Because adults more than age 65 years have more cardiac comorbidities than younger individuals, they are at increased risk for cardiac complications during ECT.[14] The ECT stimulus directly activates the vagal nerve, resulting in bradycardia or even asystole. Once the seizure is induced, there may also be sympathetic discharge, resulting in hypertension and tachycardia. In addition, parasympathetic output increases as the seizure terminates.[14,73] In the absence of cardiac comorbidities, these cardiac changes tend to be transient and benign. However, in individuals with preexisting cardiac illness they tend to be more severe, including persistent arrhythmia or, rarely, myocardial ischemia or myocardial infarction (MI).[14,74] Those at greatest risk for adverse events include individuals with recent MI, severe heart block, or arrhythmias. In addition, patients with atrial fibrillation may be at risk of embolism following ECT.[14] Medical optimization of these conditions before the procedure, including the use of β-blockers, can mitigate these risks.[15] This increased risk must be discussed with geriatric patients and weighed against the risk of not performing ECT, as part of the informed consent process.

Cerebral

Contrary to historical concerns, overwhelming evidence indicates that ECT does not cause structural damage to the brain.[14] Recent neuroimaging evidence shows remarkable neurotrophic effects of ECT.[10–12] Comorbidities that potentially increase the risk of neurologic adverse events include recent stroke, cerebral aneurysms, and amyloid angiopathy. Despite the possibility of increased risk, ECT can still be safely administered to many patients with such neurologic abnormalities, with careful hemodynamic management.[75] In the case of stroke, ECT is usually not performed until 1 to 2 months following the event, in part to allow the friable vessels to regain strength.[60] However, in cases in which ECT was emergently needed, it has been performed as soon as 4 days following stroke.[76] Despite ECT routinely causing increased blood pressure and heart rate, the number of reported serious neurologic adverse events is very small.[14,77]

Brain tumors with increased intracranial pressure pose a risk during ECT, but many patients with stable intracranial masses (such as meningiomas) without edema or associated increased intracranial pressure may be safely treated.[78]

Other Systems

Patients with serious pulmonary disease may be at increased risk from any procedure involving general anesthesia, including ECT. Airway management in patients with comorbid asthma, chronic obstructive pulmonary disease, and sleep apnea is more difficult and may result in more complications.[1] Rarely, patients aspirate during the procedure.[14]

Loose, decayed, or asymmetric teeth can be damaged during ECT because the electrical stimulus causes clenching of the jaw. Dental consultation before ECT may be prudent in cases of severe dental disease. A specially designed bite block should always be inserted to protect the patient's teeth and tongue.[14]

Comorbidities of the musculoskeletal system, including osteoporosis and spinal disk disease, may increase risk of fracture or worsening disk disease. This risk is mitigated by use of higher doses of muscle relaxant.[14] Some investigators have suggested that ECT may be an independent risk factor for falls, making fall precautions even more important in the post-ECT period.[79,80]

SUMMARY

ECT remains an essential treatment in the elderly population. It should be considered for severe and/or treatment-resistant depression, psychosis, mania, catatonia, and agitation in dementia or delirium.[1,25,33,34,38,42,49,50,59,61,63] Despite the added burden of medical illness in the geriatric population, ECT can safely be administered to most patients.[4,6–8] Cognitive effects are largely transient and patients with baseline cognitive impairment can benefit from ECT.[38,39]

REFERENCES

1. Kerner N, Prudic J. Current electroconvulsive therapy practice and research in the geriatric population. Neuropsychiatry (London) 2014;4(1):33–54.
2. Rhebergen D, Huisman A, Bouckaert F, et al. Older age is associated with rapid remission of depression after electroconvulsive therapy: a latent class growth analysis. Am J Geriatr Psychiatry 2015;23(3):274–82.
3. Rosen BH, Kung S, Lapid MI. Effect of age on psychiatric rehospitalization rates after electroconvulsive therapy for patients with depression. J ECT 2016;32(2): 93–8.
4. Kellner CH, Husain MM, Knapp RG, et al. Right unilateral ultrabrief pulse ECT in geriatric depression: phase 1 of the PRIDE study. Am J Psychiatry 2016;173(11): 1101–9.
5. Tørring N, Sanghani SN, Petrides G, et al. The mortality rate of electroconvulsive therapy: a systematic review and pooled analysis. Acta Psychiatr Scand 2017; 135(5):388–97.
6. Verwijk E, Comijs HC, Kok RM, et al. Short- and long-term neurocognitive functioning after electroconvulsive therapy in depressed elderly: a prospective naturalistic study. Int Psychogeriatr 2014;26(2):315–24.
7. Hausner L, Damian M, Sartorius A, et al. Efficacy and cognitive side effects of electroconvulsive therapy (ECT) in depressed elderly inpatients with coexisting mild cognitive impairment or dementia. J Clin Psychiatry 2011;72(1):91–7.
8. Kellner CH, Husain MM, Knapp RG, et al. A novel strategy for continuation ECT in geriatric depression: phase 2 of the PRIDE study. Am J Psychiatry 2016;173(11): 1110–8.
9. Geduldig ET, Kellner CH. Electroconvulsive therapy in the elderly: new findings in geriatric depression. Curr Psychiatry Rep 2016;18(4):1–6.
10. Wilkinson ST, Sanacora G, Bloch MH. Hippocampal volume changes following electroconvulsive therapy: a systematic review and meta-analysis. Biol Psychiatry Cogn Neurosci Neuroimaging 2017;2(4):327–35.
11. Njau S, Joshi SH, Espinoza R, et al. Neurochemical correlates of rapid treatment response to electroconvulsive therapy in patients with major depression. J Psychiatry Neurosci 2017;42(1):6–16.
12. Dukart J, Regen F, Kherif F, et al. Electroconvulsive therapy-induced brain plasticity determines therapeutic outcome in mood disorders. Proc Natl Acad Sci U S A 2014;111(3):1156–61.
13. Duma A, Pal S, Johnston J, et al. High-sensitivity cardiac troponin elevation after electroconvulsive therapy. Anesthesiology 2017;126(4):643–52.
14. Andrade C, Arumugham SS, Thirthalli J. Adverse effects of electroconvulsive therapy. Psychiatr Clin North Am 2016;39(3):513–30.
15. Bryson EO, Popeo D, Briggs M, et al. Electroconvulsive therapy (ECT) in patients with cardiac disease: hemodynamic changes. J ECT 2013;29(1):76–7.
16. Sackeim H, Malitz S. Seizure threshold in electroconvulsive therapy. Arch Gen Psychiatry 1987;44(95):355–60.

17. Gálvez V, Hadzi-Pavlovic D, Smith D, et al. Predictors of seizure threshold in right unilateral ultrabrief electroconvulsive therapy: role of concomitant medications and anaesthesia used. Brain Stimul 2015;8(3):486–92.

18. McCormick LM, Brumm MC, Benede AK, et al. Relative ineffectiveness of ultrabrief right unilateral versus bilateral electroconvulsive therapy in depression. J ECT 2009;25(4):238–42.

19. Kellner CH, Farber KG, Chen XR, et al. A systematic review of left unilateral electroconvulsive therapy. Acta Psychiatr Scand 2017;1–11.

20. Weiss AM, Hansen SM, Safranko I, et al. Effectiveness of left anterior right temporal electrode placement in electroconvulsive therapy. J ECT 2015;31(1):e1–3.

21. Bai S, Loo C, Al Abed A, et al. A computational model of direct brain excitation induced by electroconvulsive therapy: comparison among three conventional electrode placements. Brain Stimul 2012;5(3):408–21.

22. McLoughlin DM. Response to Kellner and Farber: addressing crossover of high-dose right unilateral ECT to bitemporal ECT. Am J Psychiatry 2016;173(7):731–2.

23. Fraser RM, Glass IB. Unilateral and bilateral ECT in elderly patients. A comparative study. Acta Psychiatr Scand 1980;62:13–31. Available at: http://onlinelibrary. wiley.com/o/cochrane/clcentral/articles/057/CN-00024057/frame.html.

24. Abrams R. Stimulus titration and ECT dosing. J ECT 2002;18(1):3–9.

25. Spaans HP, Sienaert P, Bouckaert F, et al. Speed of remission in elderly patients with depression: electroconvulsive therapy v. medication. Br J Psychiatry 2015; 206(1):67–71.

26. Greenberg RM. Electroconvulsive therapy: a selected review. Am J Geriatr Psychiatry 2005;13(4):268–81.

27. Oudega ML, Dols A, Adelerhof I, et al. Contribution of white matter hyperintensities, medial temporal lobe atrophy and cortical atrophy on outcome, seven to twelve years after ECT in severely depressed geriatric patients. J Affect Disord 2015;185:144–8.

28. Oudega ML, van Exel E, Wattjes MP, et al. White matter hyperintensities and cognitive impairment during electroconvulsive therapy in severely depressed elderly patients. Am J Geriatr Psychiatry 2014;22(2):157–66.

29. Oudega ML, van Exel E, Wattjes MP, et al. White matter hyperintensities, medial temporal lobe atrophy, cortical atrophy, and response to electroconvulsive therapy in severely depressed elderly patients. J Clin Psychiatry 2011;72(1):104–12.

30. Redlich R, Opel N, Grotegerd D, et al. Prediction of individual response to electroconvulsive therapy via machine learning on structural magnetic resonance imaging data. JAMA Psychiatry 2016;73(6):557.

31. van Waarde JA, Scholte HS, van Oudheusden LJB, et al. A functional MRI marker may predict the outcome of electroconvulsive therapy in severe and treatment-resistant depression. Mol Psychiatry 2015;20(5):609–14.

32. McCabe MS. ECT in the treatment of mania: a controlled study. Am J Psychiatry 1976;133(6):688–91.

33. Mukherjee S, Sackeim HA, Schnur DB. Electroconvulsive therapy of acute manic episodes: a review of 50 years' experience. Am J Psychiatry 1994;151(2):169–76. Available at: http://www.ncbi.nlm.nih.gov/pubmed/8296883. Accessed June 12, 2017.

34. Elias A, Ramalingam J, Abidi N, et al. Ultrabrief electroconvulsive therapy for mania. J ECT 2016;32(4):270–2.

35. Calabrese JR, Rapport DJ, Kimmel SE, et al. Rapid cycling bipolar disorder and its treatment with valproate. Can J Psychiatry 1993;38(3 Suppl 2):S57–61. Available at: http://www.ncbi.nlm.nih.gov/pubmed/8500080. Accessed June 19, 2017.

36. Luchini F, Lattanzi L, Bartolommei N, et al. Catatonia and neuroleptic malignant syndrome. J Nerv Ment Dis 2013;201(1):36–42.

37. Medda P, Toni C, Luchini F, et al. Catatonia in 26 patients with bipolar disorder: clinical features and response to electroconvulsive therapy. Bipolar Disord 2015;17(8):892–901.

38. Fink M, Taylor MA. Catatonia: a clinician's guide to diagnosis and treatment. New York: Cambridge University Press; 2003.

39. Weiner RD, Reti IM. Key updates in the clinical application of electroconvulsive therapy. Int Rev Psychiatry 2017;261:1–9.

40. Suzuki K, Awata S, Matsuoka H. One-year outcome after response to ECT in middle-aged and elderly patients with intractable catatonic schizophrenia. J ECT 2004;20(2):99–106.

41. Luchini F, Medda P, Mariani MG, et al. Electroconvulsive therapy in catatonic patients: efficacy and predictors of response. World J Psychiatry 2015;5(2):182–92.

42. Liu AY, Rajji TK, Blumberger DM, et al. Brain stimulation in the treatment of late-life severe mental illness other than unipolar nonpsychotic depression. Am J Geriatr Psychiatry 2014;22(3):216–40.

43. Pompili M, Lester D, Dominici G, et al. Indications for electroconvulsive treatment in schizophrenia: a systematic review. Schizophr Res 2013;146(1–3):1–9.

44. Zolezzi M. Medication management during electroconvulsant therapy. Neuropsychiatr Dis Treat 2016;12:931–9.

45. Flamarique I, Castro-Fornieles J, Garrido JM, et al. Electroconvulsive therapy and clozapine in adolescents with schizophrenia spectrum disorders. J Clin Psychopharmacol 2012;32(6):756–66.

46. Petrides G, Malur C, Braga RJ, et al. Electroconvulsive therapy augmentation in clozapine-resistant schizophrenia: a prospective, randomized study. Am J Psychiatry 2015;172(1):52–8.

47. Leyhe T, Reynolds CF, Melcher T, et al. A common challenge in older adults: classification, overlap, and therapy of depression and dementia. Alzheimers Dement 2017;13(1):59–71.

48. Dybedal GS, Tanum L, Sundet K, et al. Cognitive side-effects of electroconvulsive therapy in elderly depressed patients. Clin Neuropsychol 2014;28(7):1071–90.

49. Semkovska M, McLoughlin DM. Objective cognitive performance associated with electroconvulsive therapy for depression: a systematic review and meta-analysis. Biol Psychiatry 2010;68(6):568–77.

50. Borisovskaya A, Bryson WC, Buchholz J, et al. Electroconvulsive therapy for depression in Parkinson's disease: systematic review of evidence and recommendations. Neurodegener Dis Manag 2016;6(2):161–76.

51. Williams NR, Bentzley BS, Sahlem GL, et al. Unilateral ultra-brief pulse electroconvulsive therapy for depression in Parkinson's disease. Acta Neurol Scand 2017;135(4):407–11.

52. Rudorfer MV, Risby ED, Hsiao JK, et al. ECT alters human monoamines in a different manner from that of antidepressant drugs. Psychopharmacol Bull 1988;24(3):396–9. Available at: http://www.ncbi.nlm.nih.gov/pubmed/3153499. Accessed June 14, 2017.

53. Bolwig TG, Hertz MM, Paulson OB, et al. The permeability of the blood-brain barrier during electrically induced seizures in man. Eur J Clin Invest 1977;7(2):87–93. Available at: http://www.ncbi.nlm.nih.gov/pubmed/404164. Accessed June 14, 2017.

54. Popeo D, Kellner CH. ECT for Parkinson's disease. Med Hypotheses 2009;73(4):468–9.

55. Cumper SK, Ahle GM, Liebman LS, et al. Electroconvulsive therapy (ECT) in Parkinson's disease: ECS and dopamine enhancement. J ECT 2014;30(2):122–4.
56. Tuna Burgut F, Kellner CH. Electroconvulsive therapy (ECT) for dementia with Lewy bodies. Med Hypotheses 2010;75(2):139–40.
57. Yasui-Furukori N, Nakamura K, Katagai H, et al. The effects of electroconvulsive therapy on tardive dystonia or dyskinesia induced by psychotropic medication: a retrospective study. Neuropsychiatr Dis Treat 2014;10:1209.
58. Guo JN, Kothari JS, Leckman JF, et al. Successful treatment of Tourette syndrome with electroconvulsive therapy: a case report. Biol Psychiatry 2016;79(5):e13–4.
59. Robinson RG, Jorge RE. Post-stroke depression: a review. Am J Psychiatry 2016; 173(3):221–31.
60. Currier MB, Murray GB, Welch CC. Electroconvulsive therapy for post-stroke depressed geriatric patients. J Neuropsychiatry Clin Neurosci 1992;4(2):140–4.
61. Ujkaj M, Davidoff DA, Seiner SJ, et al. Safety and efficacy of electroconvulsive therapy for the treatment of agitation and aggression in patients with dementia. Am J Geriatr Psychiatry 2012;20(1):61–72.
62. Glass OM, Forester BP, Hermida AP. Electroconvulsive therapy (ECT) for treating agitation in dementia (major neurocognitive disorder) – a promising option. Int Psychogeriatr 2017;29(5):717–26.
63. van den Berg KS, Marijnissen RM, van Waard JA. Electroconvulsive therapy as a powerful treatment for delirium. J ECT 2016;32(1):65–6.
64. Kranaster L, Aksay SS, Bumb JM, et al. The "forgotten" treatment of alcohol withdrawal delirium with electroconvulsive therapy. Clin Neuropharmacol 2017;1. https://doi.org/10.1097/WNF.0000000000000224.
65. Tran DV, Meyer JP, Farber KG, et al. Rapid response to electroconvulsive therapy. J ECT 2017;1. https://doi.org/10.1097/YCT.0000000000000408.
66. Kellner CH. Relapse after electroconvulsive therapy (ECT). J ECT 2013;29(1):1–2.
67. van Schaik AM, Comijs HC, Sonnenberg CM, et al. Efficacy and safety of continuation and maintenance electroconvulsive therapy in depressed elderly patients: a systematic review. Am J Geriatr Psychiatry 2012;20(1):5–17.
68. O'Connor DW, Gardner B, Presnell I, et al. The effectiveness of continuation-maintenance ECT in reducing depressed older patients' hospital re-admissions. J Affect Disord 2010;120(1–3):62–6.
69. Shelef A, Mazeh D, Berger U, et al. Acute electroconvulsive therapy followed by maintenance electroconvulsive therapy decreases hospital re-admission rates of older patients with severe mental illness. J ECT 2015;31(2):125–8.
70. Bryson EO, Aloysi AS, Farber KG, et al. Individualized anesthetic management for patients undergoing electroconvulsive therapy. Anesth Analg 2017;124(6):1.
71. Nuttall GA, Bowersox MR, Douglass SB, et al. Morbidity and mortality in the use of electroconvulsive therapy. J ECT 2004;20(4):237–41.
72. Fraser LM, O'Carroll RE, Ebmeier KP. The effect of electroconvulsive therapy on autobiographical memory: a systematic review. J ECT 2008;24(1):10–7.
73. Tess AV, Smetana GW. Medical evaluation of patients undergoing electroconvulsive therapy. N Engl J Med 2009;360(14):1437–44.
74. Zielinski RJ, Roose SP, Devanand DP, et al. Cardiovascular complications of ECT in depressed patients with cardiac disease. Am J Psychiatry 1993;150(6):904–9.
75. Saito S. Anesthesia management for electroconvulsive therapy: hemodynamic and respiratory management. J Anesth 2005;19(2):142–9.
76. Alexopoulos GS, Shamoian CJ, Lucas J, et al. Medical problems of geriatric psychiatric patients and younger controls during electroconvulsive therapy. J Am

Geriatr Soc 1984;32(9):651–4. Available at: http://www.ncbi.nlm.nih.gov/pubmed/6470382. Accessed June 16, 2017.

77. Bruce BB, Henry ME, Greer DM. Ischemic stroke after electroconvulsive therapy. J ECT 2006;22(2):150–2. Available at: http://www.ncbi.nlm.nih.gov/pubmed/16801834. Accessed June 25, 2017.

78. Sajedi PI, Mitchell J, Herskovits EH, et al. Routine cross-sectional head imaging before electroconvulsive therapy: a tertiary center experience. J Am Coll Radiol 2016;13(4):429–34.

79. Rao SS, Daly JW, Sewell DD. Falls associated with electroconvulsive therapy among the geriatric population: a case report. J ECT 2008;24(2):173–5.

80. de Carle AJ, Kohn R. Electroconvulsive therapy and falls in the elderly. J ECT 2000;16(3):252–7. Available at: http://www.ncbi.nlm.nih.gov/pubmed/11005046. Accessed June 16, 2017.

81. Coffey CE, Figiel GS, Djang WT, et al. White matter hyperintensity on magnetic resonance imaging: clinical and neuroanatomic correlates in the depressed elderly. J Neuropsychiatry Clin Neurosci 1989;1(2):135–44.

82. Rubin EH, Kinscherf DA, Wehrman SA. Response to treatment of depression in the old and very old. J Geriatr Psychiatry Neurol 1991;4(2):65–70. Available at: http://www.ncbi.nlm.nih.gov/pubmed/1854423. Accessed June 21, 2017.

83. Mulsant BH, Rosen J, Thornton JE, et al. A prospective naturalistic study of electroconvulsive therapy in late-life depression. J Geriatr Psychiatry Neurol 1991;4(1):3–13. Available at: http://www.ncbi.nlm.nih.gov/pubmed/2054049. Accessed June 21, 2017.

84. Kellner CH, Monroe RR, Pritchett J, et al. Weekly ECT in geriatric depression. Convuls Ther 1992;8(4):245–52. Available at: http://www.ncbi.nlm.nih.gov/pubmed/11941174. Accessed June 21, 2017.

85. Wilkinson AM, Anderson DN, Peters S. Age and the effects of ECT. Int J Geriatr Psychiatry 1993;8(5):401–6.

86. Tomac TA, Rummans TA, Pileggi TS, et al. Safety and efficacy of electroconvulsive therapy in patients over age 85. Am J Geriatr Psychiatry 1997;5(2):126–30. Available at: http://www.ncbi.nlm.nih.gov/pubmed/9106376. Accessed June 21, 2017.

87. Tew JD, Mulsant BH, Haskett RF, et al. Acute efficacy of ECT in the treatment of major depression in the old-old. Am J Psychiatry 1999;156(12):1865–70.

88. Damm J, Eser D, Schüle C, et al. Influence of age on effectiveness and tolerability of electroconvulsive therapy. J ECT 2010;26(4):282–8.

89. Magne Bjølseth T, Engedal K, Šaltytė Benth J, et al. Speed of recovery from disorientation may predict the treatment outcome of electroconvulsive therapy (ECT) in elderly patients with major depression. J Affect Disord 2016;190:178–86.

Older Age Bipolar Disorder

Annemiek Dols, MD, PhD[a,b,c,]*, Aartjan Beekman, MD, PhD[a,b,c,d]

KEYWORDS

- Bipolar disorder • Late life • Cognition • Physical health • Somatic comorbidity
- Treatment

KEY POINTS

- Understanding of older age bipolar disorder (OABD) and recommendations for treatment can no longer simply be extrapolated from experience in mixed age groups.
- Late-onset mania has a broad differential diagnosis and requires full psychiatric and somatic work-up, including brain imaging.
- Patients with OABD require treatment adjusted to their specific characteristics and needs caused by somatic comorbidity and impaired cognitive functioning.
- Because of a shortage of controlled treatment studies in OABD, pharmacotherapy recommendations are as in adult bipolar disorder.

INTRODUCTION

Older age bipolar disorder (OABD) refers to patients older than 60 years with bipolar disorder (BD).[1,2] Of all patients with BD, 25% are older than 60 years[3] and this number is expected to increase to 50% in 2030[4] because of the aging of the total population and greater awareness of BD among older people.[5] This increase means that patients with OABD can no longer be conceptualized as a special population for whom understanding of the disorder and recommendations for treatment can simply be extrapolated from experience in mixed age groups.[6]

It was shown that the care needs of older psychiatric patients were better attended to by specialized old age psychiatry teams compared with generalized psychiatric teams,[7] indicating that strategies that are successful in younger adults cannot be extrapolated to the older patients.[8]

Disclosure: A. Beekman has received funding from the Speakers Bureau of Lundbeck. A. Dols has nothing to disclose.
[a] Department of Old Age Psychiatry, GGZinGeest and VUmc University Medical Center, Amstelveenseweg 589, 1081 JC, Amsterdam, The Netherlands; [b] Mental Health Program, Amsterdam Public Health Research Institute, Van der Boechorstsstraat 7, 1081 BT, Amsterdam, The Netherlands; [c] Mood, Anxiety and Psychosis Program, Amsterdam Neuroscience, De Boelelaan 1085, 1081 HV, Amsterdam, The Netherlands; [d] Department of Psychiatry, GGZinGeest and VUmc University Medical Center, Amstelveenseweg 589, 1081 JC, Amsterdam, The Netherlands
* Corresponding author. Department of Old Age Psychiatry, GGZinGeest and VUmc, Amstelveenseweg 589, Amsterdam 1081JC, The Netherlands.
E-mail address: a.dols@ggzingeest.nl

psych.theclinics.com

Recommendations specific for OABD regarding diagnostics, treatment, and care are warranted,[6] but most guidelines lack these specific recommendations.[9] OABD has specific aspects: somatic and psychiatric comorbidity, cognition, and age-related psychosocial functioning. These aspects define (or limit) the therapeutic options. This article discusses the diagnostic challenges in OABD and its clinical profile, somatic comorbidities, cognition, and the therapeutic options.

EPIDEMIOLOGY

Recent epidemiologic studies suggest that BD affects 0.5% to 1.0% of older adults. This percentage is lower than the prevalence of 1.4% reported in patients aged 18 to 44 years.[10,11] Patients with OABD may have been diagnosed with BD in early life and survived to old age (early onset) or become manic in later life after previous depressive episodes (converter). Approximately 10% of patients with OABD develop new-onset mania later in life, often associated with vascular changes or other brain disorders (late onset).[1,2]

Patients with OABD account for 6% of geriatric psychiatric outpatient visits and 8% to 10% of inpatient admissions,[1] with an overall prevalence of late-life mania of 6.0% in older psychiatric inpatients.[12] North American studies report that 3% of nursing home residents and 17% of older patients in psychiatric emergency rooms have BD.[1] Approximately 70% of patients with OABD are women, possibly because of increased survival rates for women.[1]

CLINICAL PROFILE

The presentation, severity, and prevalence of manic and depressive symptoms in OABD differ little from adults younger than 60 years of age[5,13] and no significant differences were found between early-onset and late-onset subtypes.[1] In most,[13,14] but not all, studies,[15,16] manic-psychotic symptoms were less frequent in OABD, in contrast with depressive episodes.[13]

AGE AT ONSET

Although there is no firmly established cutoff for early-onset BD (EOBD) versus late-onset BD (LOBD), some investigators consider age greater than or equal to 50 years as a reasonable demarcation,[1] with 5% to 17% of LOBD in OABD.[1,17] However, recently a cutoff for LOBD at 40 years was suggested to be preferred given the emerging data on subgroups with differential age at onset across the lifespan.[6] In a review on OABD, the weighted mean age of onset (manic or depressive episode) was 48.0 years (standard deviation [SD] = 6.4; range, 28–65 years) and age of onset of mania was 56.4 years (SD = 7.3; range, 38–70 years).

The clinical profile of EOBD is most often associated with a family history of mood disorder,[14,18] whereas LOBD is often associated with brain (ie, cerebrovascular) diseases,[19] a poorer response to treatment, and a higher risk of cognitive deterioration[20] or dementia.[21,22] In a previous study on OABD, no significant differences were observed in medical and psychiatric comorbidities among patients with EOBD versus LOBD,[17] possibly indicating that clinical profiles cannot be distinguished by age at onset.[23]

DIFFERENTIAL DIAGNOSES OF LATE-ONSET MANIA

Historically, mania has been defined by at least the presence of 2 symptoms (elevated mood and grandiosity) and 4 signs (hyperactivity, pressured speech, irritability, and new activities with painful consequences).[24] In the Diagnostic and Statistical Manual of Mental Disorders (DSM), Fifth Revision, the primary criteria for mania were slightly modified: "a distinct period of abnormally and persistently elevated, expansive, or irritable mood and abnormally and persistently increased activity or energy" by introducing the latter criterion.[25] Applying the new criteria may lead to a decreased prevalence of manic episodes.[26] Mania in late life is not rare; the prevalence in admitted patients is estimated at 6% with one-third of late-onset mania.[12] Whether the clinical symptom profile of late-onset mania is different from mania occurring in early adulthood is unknown.

Late-onset mania and physical health are highly linked and different hypotheses have been proposed. In general, somatic comorbidities are frequent in OABD.[27] In a retrospective study of 73 patients with mania older than 65 years, 86.3% had a somatic comorbidity.[28]

In late life, mania may occur in OABD, as a debut in patients with a previous history of recurrent depressions (late-onset mania, new-onset BD in late life), in the context of schizoaffective disorder (primary mania), or with a specific medical cause (secondary mania), as well as potentially being part of a delirium or dementia (**Table 1**).

Somatic factors may be a true cause of mania (secondary mania), or may trigger mania as a first manifestation of BD in a person with a latent vulnerability, either with or without a history of depressive episodes. However, somatic comorbidity may also be present without any causal relationship to mania. Therefore, the diagnostic work-up in late-onset mania includes full psychiatric and somatic investigation. Recommendations for diagnostic work-up in late-onset mania are summarized in **Table 2**. Several studies underline the importance of brain imaging in late-onset mania as part of the neuropsychiatric evaluation[29,30]; to study structural and subtler vascular abnormalities, MRI is preferred to computed tomography scan.

Secondary Mania

In 1978, Krauthammer and Klerman[31] introduced the concept of secondary mania as a condition with manic symptoms as a result of an underlying medical illness that could develop in people with no history of mood disorder or evidence of delirium. The list of various neurologic conditions, systemic disturbances, and medications that have been described to cause secondary mania is extensive.[32] Cerebrovascular accidents, primary or metastatic brain tumors, and traumatic brain injury have been associated with manic symptoms. Criteria for vascular mania subtype specifiers have been proposed,[33] and this concept of vascular mania seems to have some overlap with the neurologic disinhibition syndrome. Differentiating between frontal disinhibition and bipolar mania can be a challenge, because many symptoms overlap. Bipolar mania is

Table 1
Differential diagnosis of late life mania

Differential Diagnosis of Late-life Mania		
Primary mania	Late-life BD	
	Late-onset mania: new-onset BD in late life	
	Schizoaffective disorder	
Secondary mania	Caused by underlying somatic illness or medication	
	Dementia	Alzheimer disease
		Vascular dementia
		Frontotemporal dementia (behavior variant)
	Caused by underlying neurologic illness	

Table 2 Diagnostic work-up for late-onset mania	
History	Somatic and psychiatric history
	Medications, including over-the-counter medications
	History of an informant (spouse)
	Alcohol and illicit drug use
	Family history for mood illnesses
Physical examination	Including neurologic
Cognition	MMSE, full neuropsychological examination if indicated
Laboratory studies	Vitamin B, folic acid, full blood count, electrolytes, creatinine, GFR, thyroid and liver function tests
	Serum blood levels of current medications such as lithium and anticonvulsant medications
	HIV and lues serology if indicated
Imaging	MRI scan of the brain
	EEG

Abbreviations: EEG, electroencephalogram; GFR, glomerular filtration rate; HIV, human immunodeficiency virus; MMSE, Mini-Mental State Examination.

probably more characterized by elevated mood and decreased need for sleep, rather than disturbed sleep. The presence of a positive family history of affective disorder may further indicate that a somatic cause resulted in mania by triggering an existing bipolar predisposition.[31] Mania has also been linked to temporal lobe epilepsy, encephalitis, meningitis, human immunodeficiency virus encephalopathy, and tertiary syphilis.[29] In addition, thyrotoxicosis, Cushing disease, and vitamin B_{12} and niacin deficiency can produce symptoms that mimic mania.[32]

Although secondary mania can occur at any age, it is more common in older patients; this can be expected given the higher prevalence of potentially causative medical conditions and medications in late life.

Mania as a Symptom of Dementia

Mania can be a symptom of Alzheimer disease[34] or vascular dementia,[35] depending on the location of neurodegeneration. Disinhibition is also one of the core symptoms of the behavioral variant of frontotemporal dementia (bvFTD).[36] According to the recent International Consensus Criteria for bvFTD, the diagnosis is established by the presence of at least 3 of the 6 core symptoms of disinhibition, apathy, stereotyped or compulsive behavior, loss of empathy, hyperorality, and executive deficits.[36]

A possible link between frontotemporal dementia (FTD) and BD has been suggested by several case reports of patients presenting with manic symptoms as a first manifestation of bvFTD,[37,38] and patients with a lifetime diagnosis of BD evolving into bvFTD.[39,40]

There is a large clinical overlap in social cognition, executive disturbances, and behavioral profiles that might be explained by the involvement of common functional neuroanatomic networks.[41,42] A slow course with fairly normal neuroimaging has been described in a proportion of patients with bvFTD; particularly those carrying a C9orf72 repeat expansion.[43] Several case reports have shown that patients with FTD who carry this repeat expansion can present with psychiatric symptoms, including mania, years before the development of FTD.[44]

The clinical picture fulfilling criteria for possible bvFTD failing to progress over time to probable bvFTD is labeled the benign bvFTD phenocopy syndrome.[45,46] These patients show behavioral and functional impairments consistent with a frontal lobe syndrome without a progressive course and no frontal or anterior temporal atrophy or hypoperfusion with neuroimaging. Although an alternative explanation is generally lacking in these cases, it is possible that this could be an end-stage manifestation of BD.[47]

CLINICAL COURSE

The clinical course of BD is understudied in OABD. Some studies suggest there is an increasing risk of recurrence after every new episode,[48] especially among older patients,[49] with less frequent hospitalizations.[50] Because the risk of completed suicide in BD is highest for patients less than 35 years of age and EOBD is correlated significantly with suicide attempts,[51] a decreased rate of suicide in OABD would be expected and thereby they may represent a survivor cohort.[1]

Long-term outcomes of patients with BD are associated with cognitive deficits,[52,53] impaired functioning, and increased risk of dementia and premature death.[21,54] The underlying causes of this poor prognosis could include lifestyle choices, concurrent comorbidities, psychosocial adversity, and suboptimal access to health care.[55]

It is unclear whether the rate of functional recovery varies with age or whether the prevalence and presentation of rapid cycling differ between elderly and younger people,[1] but recovery rates seem to be fairly constant across affective episodes in modern treatment settings for OABD.[56]

PSYCHIATRIC COMORBIDITY

The definition of comorbidity is the occurrence of 2 syndromes in the same patient, and presupposes that they are distinct categorical entities. Psychiatric symptoms, fitting the criteria for an anxiety disorder, substance abuse, or personality disorder, may be part of BD or occur alongside it as a comorbid condition. This possibility explains why rates vary among studies, with up to 65% of bipolar patients meeting DSM-IV criteria for at least 1 comorbid axis I disorder.[57] Common psychiatric comorbidities in studies among younger adults with BD include substance abuse, anxiety disorders, attention-deficit/hyperactivity disorder, eating disorders, and personality disorders.[58] In contrast, the rates of psychiatric comorbid conditions in older adults with BD seem to be lower (anxiety disorders up to 9.8%),[17,27] except for lifetime alcohol dependence and abuse and lifetime substance dependence (lifetime substance dependence ranging from 9% to 29%). Psychiatric comorbidities in BD are associated with more severe symptoms, increased suicidality, poor adherence, and an overall more complicated course of illness.

SOMATIC COMORBIDITY

Somatic comorbidity is frequent in OABD, with an average of 3 to 4 comorbid medical conditions, including metabolic syndrome (up to 50%), hypertension (45%–69%), diabetes mellitus (18%–31%), cardiovascular disease (9%–49%), respiratory illness (4%–15%), arthritis (16%–21%), endocrine abnormalities (17%–22%),[27] as well as atopic diseases such as allergic rhinitis and asthma (6%–20%).[27,59] This burden of poor somatic health is greater than in unipolar depressed comparators,[60] and is reported to further increase with age in OABD,[61] resulting in polypharmacy[17] and decreased mean survival of 10 years.[62]

Somatic comorbidity limits treatment options for BD by drug interactions and altered drug metabolism. In OABD, screening for side effects and/or complications of medication and evaluating the patients' general physical health is recommended more frequently (2–4 times a year).[63] In patients using antipsychotics, screening for metabolic syndrome is advised (fasting lipid profile, fasting blood glucose, blood pressure, and waist circumference). Prescriptions of other doctors should be double-checked at the pharmacist, and inquiries about over-the-counter medication use are essential.

This article provides an overview of the most frequent and most important side effects of antidepressants and mood stabilizers commonly used in OABD. Because side effects are among the most important reasons for patients to stop taking their medication, careful investigation and management of these side effects is advised.[64]

Weight Gain and Metabolic Syndrome

Weight gain is a frequent and significant problem in psychiatric patients even without prescription of agents associated with metabolic syndrome. Weight gain may be caused by increased appetite, lithium-related subclinical hypothyroidism, lower metabolic rate, increased food intake secondary to improved mood, and polydipsia resulting in drinking large amounts of high-caloric drinks.[65] Antipsychotic use in older patients is associated with higher rates of hyperglycemia[66] as well as increased mortality and risk for cerebrovascular accidents.[67,68] In a recent meta-analysis the rate for metabolic syndrome in patients of all ages with schizophrenia, BD, and major depressive disorder was reported to be 32.6%[69] and higher compared with matched general population controls. Older age; higher body mass index; and use of antipsychotics, especially clozapine and olanzapine, were associated with an increased risk for metabolic syndrome. Studies of metabolic syndrome in older patients as a complication of using atypical antipsychotics are limited. In 100 older patients with schizophrenia and BD, the prevalence of metabolic syndrome was not higher than in healthy controls and not related to the use of a specific class of antipsychotics.[70] Possibly, older patients with BD who survive into old age represent a healthy survivor subpopulation.

Thyroid and Parathyroid Dysfunction

In a recent meta-analysis, lithium was associated with increased risk of endocrine side effects such as hypothyroidism and hyperparathyroidism.[71] Risk factors for development of hypothyroidism include iodine deficiency, cigarette smoking, and presence of thyroid antibodies, with women, especially younger women, and patients with diabetes at higher risk.[72] Lithium levels greater than 0.6 mmol/L were associated with increased risk for adverse effects.

Most patients are diagnosed with hypothyroidism in the first years of lithium treatment.[73] Up to 2% of lithium-treated patients require treatment with levothyroxine.[74] Monitoring of clinical symptoms provides useful guidance for treatment in addition to values of thyroid-stimulating hormone or free T4, because management of even subclinical hypothyroidism may improve outcomes among bipolar patients.[75]

In a meta-analysis of 14 observational studies a 10% increase of calcium and parathyroid hormone concentrations was found in lithium users.[71] Women aged 60 years and older were most at risk. It is recommended to measure calcium (total and adjusted) concentrations in all patients on lithium therapy at baseline and at least annually thereafter.

Kidney Failure

The effect of lithium on renal function has been the subject of several large population-based studies and meta-analyses in the past decade.[71,72,76] Rates of kidney failure seem lower that previously reported and feared, possibly as a result of modern treatment principles.[77] This article describes the 2 most common forms of kidney disease associated with lithium use: nephrogenic diabetes insipidus and chronic renal failure.

Nephrogenic diabetes insipidus is the result of lithium inhibiting the stimulating effect of antidiuretic hormone on the resorption of water in the collecting ducts of the nephron. This inhibition causes polyuria, dehydration, thirst, and compensatory polydipsia. On average, urinary concentrating ability is reduced by 15% of normal maximum after long-term lithium use[71] with a urinary production of more than 3 L a day. Other causes of polyuria and polydipsia, such as diabetes mellitus, have to be excluded as well as central diabetes insipidus and primary stimulation of the thirst center following lithium use.[78] Primary (psychogenic) polydipsia occurs predominantly in schizophrenia,[79] and dry mouth as a result of the anticholinergic side effects of drugs such as tricyclic antidepressants has to be considered.

Nephrogenic diabetes insipidus is often treated with diuretics; however, this has not been proved in placebo-controlled randomized trails.[80]

Chronic renal failure occurs in approximately 5% of all lithium users. It is not the duration of lithium use but dosing more times a day, lithium toxicities, and lithium levels more than 0.8 mmol/L that predict the occurrence of chronic renal failure.[81] Renal function is monitored by glomerular filtration rate (GFR). A recent study showed that GFR decreases with only 1.0 mL/min/1.73 m^2 each year and this was not significantly different compared with a population not using lithium (0.4 mL/min/1.73 m^2).[81]

In older patients, renal failure is more prevalent, which can be attributed to the use of supratherapeutic lithium levels, accidental intoxications, comedication (mostly diuretics and angiotensin-converting enzyme inhibitors), somatic comorbidity (mostly diabetes mellitus and hypertension), and age-related renal function decline.[81,82]

Only a very small subset of patients with stage 3 chronic renal failure progress to end-stage renal failure; the risk has been estimated to be 0.5% to 1.0%.[83,84]

Thus, especially in the large group of lithium users with only mild loss of renal function, treatable risk factors such as hypertension, hyperlipidemia, diabetes mellitus, and proteinuria have to be addressed.[77] Throughout lithium prophylaxis it is essential to monitor renal function and lithium levels at regular intervals, keeping lithium levels as low as possible, and avoid intoxication.

COGNITION

Cognitive impairment is part of BD and present in 40% to 50% of patients with OABD in the euthymic phase.[85,86] These cognitive difficulties are in the domains of attention, cognitive flexibility, processing speed, memory,[86] and fluency.[20,52]

The cognitive reserve hypothesis posits that patients with higher intelligence quotient, education, or occupational attainment have lower risks of developing dementia.[87] Cognitive reserve might be reduced because of BD or act synergistically with other neuropathologic mechanisms (eg, vascular diseases) to increase dementia risk with age.[21,56,88–90] Brain imaging in OABD shows regional gray matter atrophy and white matter hyperintensities,[91] without a pattern as seen in dementia patients but possibly a result of disease duration[92] or so-called toxic mood episodes.[93] The neuroprogression hypothesis proposing that each mood episode, especially with manic and psychotic symptoms, is neurotoxic to the brain can explain these cognitive impairment and mild brain structural changes as accelerated aging in patients with BD.[94–96]

Whether BD causes neuroprogression or even eventual dementia is not clear. Some recent studies with better methodology have confirmed the presence of significant cognitive dysfunction in euthymic patients with OABD but have not supported an increasing risk of dementia, amplification of previous cognitive dysfunction,[97–99] or faster cognitive decline in old age[97,100,101] compared with elderly without a psychiatric history after 5 years of follow-up.[102]

There is no proven effective treatment of cognitive impairment in BD; functional and cognitive remediation hold promise but have not been tested in patients with OABD.[103,104]

Risk factors for cognitive impairment are psychiatric admissions and vascular burden.[53] Cognitive impairment in OABD is associated with worse outcome.[105] There is no association between subjective cognitive complaints and cognitive impairment, urging clinicians to test cognition in OABD regardless of patients' complaints about cognition.[86,106]

TREATMENT

Caring for patients with OABD requires attention to somatic comorbidities, cognitive decline, polypharmacy, and specific phase-of-life issues, such as dealing with multiple losses, including loved ones, and occupational and social status. It is best expedited in close collaboration with their family physicians, pharmacists, and other medical specialists in order to provide comprehensive and integrated care. Systematic assessments of their needs may indicate unmet needs.[107]

Self-management and psychoeducation are the corner stones of treating BD. Empowerment and successful aging are popular terms that are meant to encourage patients to deal with their illness and feel independent of their caregivers and health professionals, and not to highlight their lack of competence while ill. Professionals need to aid patients in their self-management by providing them with knowledge about their illness (psychoeducation), insight into their illness (self-reflection), and self-interventions. A crisis management plan, including prodromal symptoms and actions to be taken, is advisable.

Psychotherapy

Existing psychosocial interventions for BD, including specific psychotherapies for OABD, have not, or have only scarcely been, studied systematically. Current practice is informed primarily by extrapolation from mixed-age studies or based on clinical experience. The Helping Older People Experience Success (HOPES) intervention was compared in a 2-year randomized trial with treatment as usual and found to improve social skills, community functioning, self-efficacy, and leisure and recreation.[108] Other psychosocial interventions hold promise for improving health and functioning in older adults with serious mental illnesses.[109] A specific psychoeducation course of approximately 12 sessions for patients with OABD and their caregivers was valued highly,[110] especially when sessions were shortened and planned during daytime.

Specific Pharmacotherapies

Research on pharmacotherapy in OABD is limited because older adults are often excluded from randomized controlled registration trials because of the increasing risk of medical complications with advancing age. Most guidelines recommend that first-line treatment of OABD should be similar to that of BD, with specific attention to vulnerability to side effects and somatic comorbidity.[9] In the report of the OABD Task Force of the International Society for Bipolar Disorders, the available studies (including mixed-age samples) are discussed.[6] This article summarizes the pharmacotherapeutic recommendations for each phase of BD.

Mania

For acute bipolar mania, lithium is the first choice in OABD, but there is also limited evidence for the efficacy of antipsychotics. In a network analysis, carbamazepine, valproate, haloperidol, lithium, olanzapine, quetiapine, and risperidone were more effective than placebo in adult BD[111]; haloperidol was most effective. It is recommended in the acute phase to choose a medication that can be continued in the maintenance phase. Sleep disturbance and agitation can be treated with benzodiazepines temporarily.

Bipolar depression

In a network analysis, lurasidone, valproate, quetiapine, and the combinations of fluoxetine with olanzapine, and olanzapine and lamotrigine were significantly more effective than placebo for the treatment of bipolar depression in adult BD.[112]

The use of antidepressants in BD remains controversial because of limited proof for effectiveness[113]; moreover, tricyclic antidepressants and venlafaxine are associated with increased risk of triggering mania (known as switching).

Maintenance treatment

In a systematic review, lithium was found to be most effective for long-term treatment of adult BD by reducing relapse of mania and depression and suicide risk.[114,115] Olanzapine or quetiapine can be considered as second choices.

Prescribing Lithium in Older Age Bipolar Disorder

Therapeutic serum levels can be achieved with a 25% to 50% lower dose compared with younger adults.[3] Lithium serum levels of 0.4 to 0.6 mmol/L can be effective, although levels of 0.8 mmol/L or higher may be needed for therapeutic efficacy. Balancing toxicity and clinical efficacy is a great challenge when using lithium for the treatment of older adults with BD. In general, there is a trend for underuse of lithium, most pronounced in North America,[116] although the alternative medication (anticonvulsants, antipsychotics, antidepressants, and benzodiazepines) have an even more pronounced and disturbing paucity of information on efficacy and side effects in older patients.

Electroconvulsive therapy

The effectiveness of electroconvulsive therapy (ECT) has been shown in BD[117] for both manic and depressive symptoms. For treatment-resistant bipolar depression, ECT is the treatment option with the most evidence.[118] Nevertheless, in most guidelines, ECT is offered only as second-line or third-line treatment of refractory depression, possibly because of stigma and concern for cognitive side effects. There are no systematic studies on the effectiveness of ECT in older patients with BD. However, extrapolating results of ECT in younger adults with BD[117] and older adults with unipolar disorder,[119] a superior effect of ECT in older patients with BD can be expected in the acute phases (mania, depression, and mixed episode), most specific in cases of pharmacotherapy resistance, previous ECT response, or urgent safety concerns (severe suicidality, physical exhaustion, or refusal of all foods and fluids).

Cognitive side effects of ECT have been studied in older patients with unipolar depression,[120] and postictal confusion has been described but most studies report improvements of cognitive functions after ECT, most likely caused by recovery of depressed mood, concentration, and attention. As was concluded in an expert consensus paper, ECT remains an important treatment option in OABD.[6]

SUMMARY

Older patients with BD are vulnerable and require treatment adjusted to their specific characteristics and needs caused by somatic comorbidity and impaired cognitive functioning.

OABD is understudied and most knowledge and recommendations about OABD are based on studies in younger or mixed age groups. Because findings in younger adults with BD cannot be extrapolated to OABD, more research in OABD is warranted.

REFERENCES

1. Depp CA, Jeste DV. Bipolar disorder in older adults: a critical review. Bipolar Disord 2004;6(5):343–67.
2. Sajatovic M, Kessing L. Bipolar disorder in older adults: a critical review. In: Yatham LN, Maj M, editors. Bipolar disorder - clinical and neurobiological foundations. Singapore: Markono Print Media; 2010.
3. Sajatovic M, Gyulai L, Calabrese JR, et al. Maintenance treatment outcomes in older patients with bipolar I disorder. Am J Geriatr Psychiatry 2005;13(4): 305–11.
4. Jeste DV, Alexopoulos GS, Bartels SJ, et al. Consensus statement on the upcoming crisis in geriatric mental health: research agenda for the next 2 decades. Arch Gen Psychiatry 1999;56(9):848–53.
5. Almeida OP, Fenner S. Bipolar disorder: similarities and differences between patients with illness onset before and after 65 years of age. Int Psychogeriatr 2002; 14(3):311–22.
6. Sajatovic M, Strejilevich SA, Gildengers AG, et al. A report on older-age bipolar disorder from the International Society for Bipolar Disorders Task Force. Bipolar Disord 2015;17(7):689–704.
7. Abdul-Hamid WK, Lewis-Cole K, Holloway F, et al. Comparision of how old age psychiatry and general adult psychiatry services meet the needs of elderly people with functional mental illness: cross-sectional survey. Br J Psychiatry 2015; 207(5):440–3.
8. Warner JP. Old age psychiatry in the modern age. Br J Psychiatry 2015;207(5): 375–6.
9. Dols A, Kessing LV, Strejilevich SA, et al. Do current national and international guidelines have specific recommendations for older adults with bipolar disorder? A brief report. Int J Geriatr Psychiatry 2016;31(12):1295–300.
10. Hirschfeld RM, Calabrese JR, Weissman MM, et al. Screening for bipolar disorder in the community. J Clin Psychiatry 2003;64(1):53–9.
11. Kessler RC, Berglund P, Demler O, et al. Lifetime prevalence and age-of-onset distributions of DSM-IV disorders in the National Comorbidity Survey Replication. Arch Gen Psychiatry 2005;62(6):593–602.
12. Dols A, Kupka RW, van Lammeren A, et al. The prevalence of late-life mania: a review. Bipolar Disord 2014;16(2):113–8.
13. Kessing LV. Diagnostic subtypes of bipolar disorder in older versus younger adults. Bipolar Disord 2006;8(1):56–64.
14. Schurhoff F, Bellivier F, Jouvent R, et al. Early and late onset bipolar disorders: two different forms of manic-depressive illness? J Affect Disord 2000;58(3): 215–21.
15. Depp CA, Jin H, Mohamed S, et al. Bipolar disorder in middle-aged and elderly adults: is age of onset important? J Nerv Ment Dis 2004;192(11):796–9.

16. Ernst CL, Goldberg JF. Clinical features related to age at onset in bipolar disorder. J Affect Disord 2004;82(1):21–7.

17. Dols A, Rhebergen D, Beekman A, et al. Psychiatric and medical comorbidities: results from a bipolar elderly cohort study. Am J Geriatr Psychiatry 2014;22(11): 1066–74.

18. Thesing CS, Stek ML, van Grootheest DS, et al. Childhood abuse, family history and stressors in older patients with bipolar disorder in relation to age at onset. J Affect Disord 2015;184:249–55.

19. Cassidy F, Carroll BJ. Vascular risk factors in late onset mania. Psychol Med 2002;32(2):359–62.

20. Schouws SN, Comijs HC, Stek ML, et al. Cognitive impairment in early and late bipolar disorder. Am J Geriatr Psychiatry 2009;17(6):508–15.

21. Kessing LV, Andersen PK. Does the risk of developing dementia increase with the number of episodes in patients with depressive disorder and in patients with bipolar disorder? J Neurol Neurosurg Psychiatry 2004;75(12):1662–6.

22. Almeida OP, McCaul K, Hankey GJ, et al. Risk of dementia and death in community-dwelling older men with bipolar disorder. Br J Psychiatry 2016; 209(2):121–6.

23. Joslyn C, Hawes DJ, Hunt C, et al. Is age of onset associated with severity, prognosis, and clinical features in bipolar disorder? A meta-analytic review. Bipolar Disord 2016;18(5):389–403.

24. Kendler KS. The clinical features of mania and their representation in modern diagnostic criteria. Psychol Med 2016;1–17.

25. Diagnostic and Statistical Manual of Mental Disorders. 5th edition. Washington, DC: American Psychiatric Association; 2013.

26. Machado-Vieira R, Luckenbaugh DA, Ballard ED, et al. Increased activity or energy as a primary criterion for the diagnosis of bipolar mania in DSM-5: findings from the STEP-BD study. Am J Psychiatry 2017;174(1):70–6.

27. Lala SV, Sajatovic M. Medical and psychiatric comorbidities among elderly individuals with bipolar disorder: a literature review. J Geriatr Psychiatry Neurol 2012;25(1):20–5.

28. Lehmann SW, Rabins PV. Factors related to hospitalization in elderly manic patients with early and late-onset bipolar disorder. Int J Geriatr Psychiatry 2006; 21(11):1060–4.

29. Brooks JO 3rd, Hoblyn JC. Secondary mania in older adults. Am J Psychiatry 2005;162(11):2033–8.

30. Arciniegas DB. New-onset bipolar disorder in late life: a case of mistaken identity. Am J Psychiatry 2006;163(2):198–203.

31. Krauthammer C, Klerman GL. Secondary mania: manic syndromes associated with antecedent physical illness or drugs. Arch Gen Psychiatry 1978;35(11): 1333–9.

32. Van Gerpen MW, Johnson JE, Winstead DK. Mania in the geriatric patient population: a review of the literature. Am J Geriatr Psychiatry 1999;7(3):188–202.

33. Steffens DC, Krishnan KR. Structural neuroimaging and mood disorders: recent findings, implications for classification, and future directions. Biol Psychiatry 1998;43(10):705–12.

34. Woodward M, Jacova C, Black SE, et al. Differentiating the frontal variant of Alzheimer's disease. Int J Geriatr Psychiatry 2010;25(7):732–8.

35. Staekenborg SS, Su T, van Straaten EC, et al. Behavioural and psychological symptoms in vascular dementia; differences between small- and large-vessel disease. J Neurol Neurosurg Psychiatry 2010;81(5):547–51.

36. Rascovsky K, Hodges JR, Knopman D, et al. Sensitivity of revised diagnostic criteria for the behavioural variant of frontotemporal dementia. Brain 2011; 134(Pt 9):2456–77.

37. Vorspan F, Bertoux M, Brichant-Petitjean C, et al. Relapsing-remitting behavioural variant of frontotemporal dementia in a bipolar patient. Funct Neurol 2012; 27(3):193–6.

38. Kerstein AH, Schroeder RW, Baade LE, et al. Frontotemporal dementia mimicking bipolar disorder. J Psychiatr Pract 2013;19(6):498–500.

39. Cerami C, Marcone A, Galimberti D, et al. From genotype to phenotype: two cases of genetic frontotemporal lobar degeneration with premorbid bipolar disorder. J Alzheimers Dis 2011;27(4):791–7.

40. Pavlovic A, Marley J, Sivakumar V. Development of frontotemporal dementia in a case of bipolar affective disorder: is there a link? BMJ Case Rep 2011;2011 [pii: bcr0920103303].

41. Zhou J, Seeley WW. Network dysfunction in Alzheimer's disease and frontotemporal dementia: implications for psychiatry. Biol Psychiatry 2014;75(7):565–73.

42. Lois G, Linke J, Wessa M. Altered functional connectivity between emotional and cognitive resting state networks in euthymic bipolar I disorder patients. PLoS One 2014;9(10):e107829.

43. Khan BK, Yokoyama JS, Takada LT, et al. Atypical, slowly progressive behavioural variant frontotemporal dementia associated with C9ORF72 hexanucleotide expansion. J Neurol Neurosurg Psychiatry 2012;83(4):358–64.

44. Meisler MH, Grant AE, Jones JM, et al. C9ORF72 expansion in a family with bipolar disorder. Bipolar Disord 2013;15(3):326–32.

45. Kipps CM, Hodges JR, Hornberger M. Nonprogressive behavioural frontotemporal dementia: recent developments and clinical implications of the 'bvFTD phenocopy syndrome'. Curr Opin Neurol 2010;23(6):628–32.

46. Gossink FT, Dols A, Kerssens CJ, et al. Psychiatric diagnoses underlying the phenocopy syndrome of behavioural variant frontotemporal dementia. J Neurol Neurosurg Psychiatry 2015;87(1):64–8.

47. Dols A, Krudop W, Moller C, et al. Late life bipolar disorder evolving into frontotemporal dementia mimic. Neuropsychiatr Dis Treat 2016;12:2207–12.

48. Kessing LV. Recurrence in affective disorder. II. Effect of age and gender. Br J Psychiatry 1998;172:29–34.

49. Angst J, Preisig M. Course of a clinical cohort of unipolar, bipolar and schizoaffective patients. Results of a prospective study from 1959 to 1985. Schweiz Arch Neurol Psychiatr (1985) 1995;146(1):5–16.

50. Kessing LV, Hansen MG, Andersen PK. Course of illness in depressive and bipolar disorders. Naturalistic study, 1994-1999. Br J Psychiatry 2004;185:372–7.

51. Schaffer A, Isometsä ET, Tondo L, et al. International Society for Bipolar Disorders Task Force on Suicide: meta-analyses and meta-regression of correlates of suicide attempts and suicide deaths in bipolar disorder. Bipolar Disord 2015;17(1):1–16.

52. Samame C, Martino DJ, Strejilevich SA. A quantitative review of neurocognition in euthymic late-life bipolar disorder. Bipolar Disord 2013;15(6):633–44.

53. Schouws SN, Stek ML, Comijs HC, et al. Risk factors for cognitive impairment in elderly bipolar patients. J Affect Disord 2010;125(1–3):330–5.

54. Almeida OP, Hankey GJ, Yeap BB, et al. Mortality among people with severe mental disorders who reach old age: a longitudinal study of a community-representative sample of 37,892 men. PLoS One 2014;9(10):e111882.

55. Almeida OP. Does bipolar disorder have a benign course? Int Psychogeriatr 2016;28(11):1755-7.
56. Kessing LV, Mortensen PB. Recovery from episodes during the course of affective disorder: a case-register study. Acta Psychiatr Scand 1999;100(4):279-87.
57. McElroy SL, Altshuler LL, Suppes T, et al. Axis I psychiatric comorbidity and its relationship to historical illness variables in 288 patients with bipolar disorder. Am J Psychiatry 2001;158(3):420-6.
58. Krishnan KR. Psychiatric and medical comorbidities of bipolar disorder. Psychosom Med 2005;67(1):1-8.
59. Tsai SY, Kuo CJ, Chung KH, et al. Cognitive dysfunction and medical morbidity in elderly outpatients with bipolar disorder. Am J Geriatr Psychiatry 2009;17(12): 1004-11.
60. Gildengers AG, Whyte EM, Drayer RA, et al. Medical burden in late-life bipolar and major depressive disorders. Am J Geriatr Psychiatry 2008;16(3):194-200.
61. Fenn HH, Bauer MS, Altshuler L, et al. Medical comorbidity and health-related quality of life in bipolar disorder across the adult age span. J Affect Disord 2005;86(1):47-60.
62. Westman J, Hallgren J, Wahlbeck K, et al. Cardiovascular mortality in bipolar disorder: a population-based cohort study in Sweden. BMJ Open 2013;3(4) [pii:e002373].
63. Ng F, Mammen OK, Wilting I, et al. The International Society for Bipolar Disorders (ISBD) consensus guidelines for the safety monitoring of bipolar disorder treatments. Bipolar Disord 2009;11(6):559-95.
64. Dols A, Sienaert P, van Gerven H, et al. The prevalence and management of side effects of lithium and anticonvulsants as mood stabilizers in bipolar disorder from a clinical perspective: a review. Int Clin Psychopharmacol 2013;28(6): 287-96.
65. Torrent C, Amann B, Sanchez-Moreno J, et al. Weight gain in bipolar disorder: pharmacological treatment as a contributing factor. Acta Psychiatr Scand 2008;118(1):4-18.
66. Lipscombe LL, Levesque L, Gruneir A, et al. Antipsychotic drugs and hyperglycemia in older patients with diabetes. Arch Intern Med 2009;169(14):1282-9.
67. Setoguchi S, Wang PS, Alan Brookhart M, et al. Potential causes of higher mortality in elderly users of conventional and atypical antipsychotic medications. J Am Geriatr Soc 2008;56(9):1644-50.
68. Wang PS, Schneeweiss S, Avorn J, et al. Risk of death in elderly users of conventional vs. atypical antipsychotic medications. N Engl J Med 2005;353(22): 2335-41.
69. Vancampfort D, Stubbs B, Mitchell AJ, et al. Risk of metabolic syndrome and its components in people with schizophrenia and related psychotic disorders, bipolar disorder and major depressive disorder: a systematic review and meta-analysis. World Psychiatry 2015;14(3):339-47.
70. Konz HW, Meesters PD, Paans NP, et al. Screening for metabolic syndrome in older patients with severe mental illness. Am J Geriatr Psychiatry 2014;22(11): 1116-20.
71. McKnight RF, Adida M, Budge K, et al. Lithium toxicity profile: a systematic review and meta-analysis. Lancet 2012;379(9817):721-8.
72. Shine B, McKnight RF, Leaver L, et al. Long-term effects of lithium on renal, thyroid, and parathyroid function: a retrospective analysis of laboratory data. Lancet 2015;386(9992):461-8.

73. van Melick EJ, Wilting I, Meinders AE, et al. Prevalence and determinants of thyroid disorders in elderly patients with affective disorders: lithium and nonlithium patients. Am J Geriatr Psychiatry 2010;18(5):395–403.

74. Kirov G, Tredget J, John R, et al. A cross-sectional and a prospective study of thyroid disorders in lithium-treated patients. J Affect Disord 2005;87(2–3):313–7.

75. Najafi L, Malek M, Hadian A, et al. Depressive symptoms in patients with subclinical hypothyroidism–the effect of treatment with levothyroxine: a double-blind randomized clinical trial. Endocr Res 2015;40(3):121–6.

76. Kessing LV, Gerds TA, Feldt-Rasmussen B, et al. Use of lithium and anticonvulsants and the rate of chronic kidney disease: a nationwide population-based study. JAMA Psychiatry 2015;72(12):1182–91.

77. Aiff H, Attman PO, Aurell M, et al. The impact of modern treatment principles may have eliminated lithium-induced renal failure. J Psychopharmacol 2014; 28(2):151–4.

78. Cox M, Singer I. Lithium and water metabolism. Am J Med 1975;59(2):153–7.

79. Mercier-Guidez E, Loas G. Polydipsia: review of the literature. Encephale 1998; 24(3):223–9 [in French].

80. Bedford JJ, Weggery S, Ellis G, et al. Lithium-induced nephrogenic diabetes insipidus: renal effects of amiloride. Clin J Am Soc Nephrol 2008;3(5):1324–31.

81. Clos S, Rauchhaus P, Severn A, et al. Long-term effect of lithium maintenance therapy on estimated glomerular filtration rate in patients with affective disorders: a population-based cohort study. Lancet Psychiatry 2015;2(12):1075–83.

82. Rej S, Herrmann N, Shulman K. The effects of lithium on renal function in older adults–a systematic review. J Geriatr Psychiatry Neurol 2012;25(1):51–61.

83. Tredget J, Kirov A, Kirov G. Effects of chronic lithium treatment on renal function. J Affect Disord 2010;126(3):436–40.

84. Bendz H, Schon S, Attman PO, et al. Renal failure occurs in chronic lithium treatment but is uncommon. Kidney Int 2010;77(3):219–24.

85. Gildengers AG, Butters MA, Seligman K, et al. Cognitive functioning in late-life bipolar disorder. Am J Psychiatry 2004;161(4):736–8.

86. Schouws SN, Comijs HC, Stek ML, et al. Self-reported cognitive complaints in elderly bipolar patients. Am J Geriatr Psychiatry 2012;20(8):700–6.

87. Stern Y. What is cognitive reserve? Theory and research application of the reserve concept. J Int Neuropsychol Soc 2002;8(3):448–60.

88. da Silva J, Goncalves-Pereira M, Xavier M, et al. Affective disorders and risk of developing dementia: systematic review. Br J Psychiatry 2013;202(3):177–86.

89. Meng X, D'Arcy C. Education and dementia in the context of the cognitive reserve hypothesis: a systematic review with meta-analyses and qualitative analyses. PLoS One 2012;7(6):e38268.

90. Wu KY, Chang CM, Liang HY, et al. Increased risk of developing dementia in patients with bipolar disorder: a nested matched case-control study. Bipolar Disord 2013;15(7):787–94.

91. Vederine FE, Wessa M, Leboyer M, et al. A meta-analysis of whole-brain diffusion tensor imaging studies in bipolar disorder. Prog Neuropsychopharmacol Biol Psychiatry 2011;35(8):1820–6.

92. Gildengers AG, Chung KH, Huang SH, et al. Neuroprogressive effects of lifetime illness duration in older adults with bipolar disorder. Bipolar Disord 2014;16(6): 617–23.

93. Berk M, Kapczinski F, Andreazza AC, et al. Pathways underlying neuroprogression in bipolar disorder: focus on inflammation, oxidative stress and neurotrophic factors. Neurosci Biobehav Rev 2010;35(3):804–17.

94. Rizzo LB, Costa LG, Mansur RB, et al. The theory of bipolar disorder as an illness of accelerated aging: implications for clinical care and research. Neurosci Biobehav Rev 2014;42:157–69.
95. Berk M, Hallam KT, McGorry PD. The potential utility of a staging model as a course specifier: a bipolar disorder perspective. J Affect Disord 2007; 100(1–3):279–81.
96. Kapczinski F, Dias VV, Kauer-Sant'Anna M, et al. Clinical implications of a staging model for bipolar disorders. Expert Rev Neurother 2009;9(7):957–66.
97. Delaloye C, Moy G, de Bilbao F, et al. Longitudinal analysis of cognitive performances and structural brain changes in late-life bipolar disorder. Int J Geriatr Psychiatry 2011;26(12):1309–18.
98. Depp CA, Savla GN, Moore DJ, et al. Short-term course of neuropsychological abilities in middle-aged and older adults with bipolar disorder. Bipolar Disord 2008;10(6):684–90.
99. Martino DJ, Strejilevich SA, Marengo E, et al. Relationship between neurocognitive functioning and episode recurrences in bipolar disorder. J Affect Disord 2013;147(1–3):345–51.
100. Schouws SN, Stek ML, Comijs HC, et al. Cognitive decline in elderly bipolar disorder patients: a follow-up study. Bipolar Disord 2012;14(7):749–55.
101. Gildengers AG, Chisholm D, Butters MA, et al. Two-year course of cognitive function and instrumental activities of daily living in older adults with bipolar disorder: evidence for neuroprogression? Psychol Med 2013;43(4):801–11.
102. Schouws SN, Comijs HC, Dols A, et al. Five-year follow-up of cognitive impairment in older adults with bipolar disorder. Bipolar Disord 2016;18(2):148–54.
103. Demant KM, Vinberg M, Kessing LV, et al. Effects of short-term cognitive remediation on cognitive dysfunction in partially or fully remitted individuals with bipolar disorder: results of a randomised controlled trial. PLoS One 2015;10(6): e0127955.
104. Torrent C, Bonnin Cdel M, Martínez-Arán A, et al. Efficacy of functional remediation in bipolar disorder: a multicenter randomized controlled study. Am J Psychiatry 2013;170(8):852–9.
105. Burdick KE, Goldberg JF, Harrow M. Neurocognitive dysfunction and psychosocial outcome in patients with bipolar I disorder at 15-year follow-up. Acta Psychiatr Scand 2010;122(6):499–506.
106. Demant KM, Vinberg M, Kessing LV, et al. Assessment of subjective and objective cognitive function in bipolar disorder: correlations, predictors and the relation to psychosocial function. Psychiatry Res 2015;229(1–2):565–71.
107. Dautzenberg G, Lans L, Meesters PD, et al. The care needs of older patients with bipolar disorder. Aging Ment Health 2016;20(9):899–907.
108. Mueser KT, Pratt SI, Bartels SJ, et al. Randomized trial of social rehabilitation and integrated health care for older people with severe mental illness. J Consult Clin Psychol 2010;78(4):561–73.
109. Bartels SJ, Pratt SI. Psychosocial rehabilitation and quality of life for older adults with serious mental illness: recent findings and future research directions. Curr Opin Psychiatry 2009;22(4):381–5.
110. Colom F, Vieta E, Martinez-Aran A, et al. A randomized trial on the efficacy of group psychoeducation in the prophylaxis of recurrences in bipolar patients whose disease is in remission. Arch Gen Psychiatry 2003;60(4):402–7.
111. Cipriani A, Barbui C, Salanti G, et al. Comparative efficacy and acceptability of antimanic drugs in acute mania: a multiple-treatments meta-analysis. Lancet 2011;378(9799):1306–15.

112. Bipolar disorder: assessment and management. Clinical guideline [CG185]. 2017. Available at: nice.org.uk/guidance/cg185. Accessed November 24, 2017.

113. Pacchiarotti I, Bond DJ, Baldessarini RJ, et al. The International Society for Bipolar Disorders (ISBD) task force report on antidepressant use in bipolar disorders. Am J Psychiatry 2013;170(11):1249–62.

114. Cipriani A, Hawton K, Stockton S, et al. Lithium in the prevention of suicide in mood disorders: updated systematic review and meta-analysis. BMJ 2013; 346:f3646.

115. Geddes JR, Burgess S, Hawton K, et al. Long-term lithium therapy for bipolar disorder: systematic review and meta-analysis of randomized controlled trials. Am J Psychiatry 2004;161(2):217–22.

116. Carney SM, Goodwin GM. Lithium - a continuing story in the treatment of bipolar disorder. Acta Psychiatr Scand Suppl 2005;(426):7–12.

117. Versiani M, Cheniaux E, Landeira-Fernandez J. Efficacy and safety of electroconvulsive therapy in the treatment of bipolar disorder: a systematic review. J ECT 2010;27(2):153–64.

118. Sienaert P, Lambrichts L, Dols A, et al. Evidence-based treatment strategies for treatment-resistant bipolar depression: a systematic review. Bipolar Disord 2012;15(1):61–9.

119. Wurff Van der FFB, Stek ML, Hoogendijk WL, et al. Electroconvulsive therapy for the depressed elderly. Cochrane Database Syst Rev 2003;2:CD003593.

120. Tielkes CE, Comijs HC, Verwijk E, et al. The effects of ECT on cognitive functioning in the elderly: a review. Int J Geriatr Psychiatry 2008;23(8):789–95.

Neurologic Changes and Depression

Ryan D. Greene, Psy D[a,b,*], Sophia Wang, MD[a,b,c,d]

KEYWORDS

- Major depressive disorder • Subjective cognitive impairment
- Mild cognitive impairment • Neurocognitive disorder • Neuropsychological testing
- Neuroimaging • Psychotherapy • Antidepressants

KEY POINTS

- The assessment of late-life depression with comorbid cognitive impairment can be challenging and requires a clear clinical history and a thorough medical and cognitive assessment.
- There are several neuropsychological changes associated with late-life depression, ranging from subjective cognitive complaints to mild cognitive impairment to dementia.
- Changes on neuroimaging and in several biomarkers (eg, apolipoprotein E e4 allele, beta-amyloid, tau, neurotrophins, and so forth) have been associated with late-life depression.
- Multiple psychotherapeutic techniques have been found effective in the treatment of late-life depression as well as holistic/nontraditional, pharmacologic, and brain-stimulation approaches.

INTRODUCTION

Late-life depression affects 3.0% to 4.5% adults older than 65 years in the United States.[1] For many older adults with depression, affective symptoms are accompanied by cognitive difficulties, which can range from subjective cognitive complaints to mild cognitive impairment (MCI) to dementia. Epidemiologic findings suggest that late-life depression may be a risk factor for dementia.[2,3] Given the relatively high prevalence of depression in older adults and a growing focus on modifiable risk factors for dementia, there is interest in better understanding the complex relationship between depression and cognitive impairment. This review focuses on individuals with unipolar depression without psychotic features with comorbid MCI or dementia. To align with the

Disclosure Statement: S. Wang receives grant support from NIA (#2P30AG010133). R. Greene has nothing to disclose.

[a] Richard L. Roudebush VAMC, 1481 W. 10th Street, Indianapolis, IN 46202, USA; [b] Department of Pyschiatry, Indiana University School of Medicine, Goodman Campbell Neuroscience Center, 355 W. 16th Street, Indianapolis, IN 46202, USA; [c] Center of Health Innovation and Implementation Science, Center for Translational Science and Innovation, Indianapolis, IN, USA; [d] Sandra Eskenazi Center for Brain Care Innovation, Eskenazi Hospital, Indianapolis, IN, USA
* Corresponding author.
E-mail address: rygreene@iupui.edu

Psychiatr Clin N Am 41 (2018) 111–126
https://doi.org/10.1016/j.psc.2017.10.009
0193-953X/18/Published by Elsevier Inc.

psych.theclinics.com

terminology used in earlier literature and within the *International Classification of Diseases, Tenth Revision* coding system, the authors use *Diagnostic and Statistical Manual of Mental Disorder* (Fourth Edition, Text Revision) (*DSM-IV TR*) terminology (ie, MCI and dementia) instead of the *DSM-5* terminology for neurocognitive disorders.

Clinical Assessment of Late-Life Depression with Comorbid Cognitive Impairment

Accurately diagnosing late-life depression can be challenging because of the wide variety of symptom presentations.[4] A few key points can guide the clinical evaluation of depression in older adults with comorbid cognitive impairment. Specifically, these are (1) receiving a detailed history from both the patients and their informants, (2) following patients longitudinally to monitor symptom progression, and (3) interviewing with potential reversible causes of cognitive impairment in mind (eg, substance use, metabolic problems, and so forth).

First, the most powerful diagnostic tool the clinician has is the clinical interview. Obtaining a detailed history from both the patients and their informants will be a critical piece to determine whether the patients have a primary mood and/or cognitive disorder. In certain cases, a detailed neuropsychological evaluation may be necessary to delineate cognitive and mood symptoms. Furthermore, neuropsychological testing is indicated when there are questions of multiple comorbidities, questionable self- or informant-report, and to establish a baseline in mild dementia and MCI cases. An accurate informant can be especially helpful, as many patients frequently experience anosognosia (lack of awareness due to neurologic disease) about their cognitive deficits or alexithymia (inability to describe one's feelings). Patients may also experience variations in their mood depending on the time of day (ie, diurnal variations); therefore, an informant may be helpful in mapping the overall mood.

Second, clinicians can follow patients' symptoms over time. This technique can be important in the diagnosis of more complex cases when it is difficult to determine whether patients' have primary cognitive disorder, primary mood disorder, or both. Clinicians should determine whether emotional and cognitive symptoms resolve, remain static, or progress over time. For example, if the cognitive symptoms worsen despite stable or improved mood, this would suggest a primary cognitive disorder. Alternatively, if the cognitive symptoms vary with emotional state, for example, worsening with increased emotional distress, this would suggest a primary mood disorder.

When patients present with both significant emotional and cognitive complaints, clinicians should aggressively treat the depressive symptoms first and then reassess cognitive symptoms after some resolution of the severe emotional distress. Literature has indicated that mild to moderate depression is best treated with a combination of antidepressants and psychotherapy.[5] However, the patients' cognitive capacity to engage in psychotherapy should always be considered. Electroconvulsive therapy (ECT) and other brain-stimulation therapies are generally reserved for severe or treatment-resistant cases.

Third, clinicians should always approach these complex cases considering potential reversible causes of the patients' mood and cognitive symptoms. One of the most overlooked, but easily reversible, causes of cognitive impairment in older adults is medication side effects. Specifically, research has shown that benzodiazepines, anticholinergics, opiates, non-narcotic pain medications (ie, tramadol), hypnotics, and antipsychotics have been associated with cognitive symptoms.[6] Substance use in older adults is frequently not explored thoroughly, particularly in regard to alcohol and cannabis use.[7] Finally, a thorough workup for late-life depression should also include a comprehensive laboratory workup, assessing hematologic, metabolic, toxic, and infectious contributions to cognitive and/or affective symptoms.

Risk Factors

The interactions between medical illnesses, depression, and cognitive impairments are typically multidirectional, making it difficult to distinguish causes of current symptom presentations. Men, Caucasians, and individuals with functional impairments were more likely to present with affective symptoms of depression in MCI and early Alzheimer disease (AD).[8] Cerebrovascular disease has been associated with both late-life depression and comorbid executive dysfunction.[9,10] Cognition and mood can also be impacted by other causes of organ failure, including chronic renal failure[11,12] and chronic obstructive pulmonary disease.[13,14]

SUICIDE AND COGNITION

The incidence of suicide among individuals aged 85 years and older in the United States is 17.8 deaths per 100,000 (compared with 15.0 deaths per 100,000 for those aged 65–84 years).[15] Although aging alone may increase the suicide risk, further research is needed to clarify the relationship between cognitive changes from aging and suicidality. The ventromedial prefrontal cortices, which are important in reasoning and decision-making, may become impaired in later adulthood[16] and consequently increase the risk for suicidality. This impairment may be further exacerbated by changes in social support, that is, depressed elders with suicide attempts tend to have greater difficulties socially.[17] Finally, many medical illnesses affecting older adults are often accompanied by comorbid depression and cognitive impairments, likely predisposing the affected older adult to suicidality.[11,18,19]

NEUROPSYCHOLOGICAL CHANGES IN DEPRESSION
Cognitive Aging

Cognitive aging is characterized by gradual changes in cognitive functioning associated with normal aging.[20] These changes can be variable between patients, are not secondary to a neurodegenerative illness or typically accompanied by functional decline, and generally accelerate in late life. Specific cognitive changes associated with aging include trouble with memory recall and executive dysfunction and slowed processing speed. In contrast, visuospatial skills, crystallized intelligence, and vocabulary knowledge remain stable.[21] Generally, good management of multiple health factors, including hypertension, diabetes, chronic obstructive pulmonary disease, and so forth, and psychiatric disorders (including depression and anxiety) can help mitigate some of the changes associated with normal aging.

Subjective Cognitive Impairment and Depression

Subjective cognitive impairment (SCI) refers to the perception of cognitive decline without evidence of deficits on objective measures.[22] Several cross-sectional studies on the relationship between subjective cognitive complaints and objective impairments on cognitive testing have shown conflicting findings, ranging from a positive correlation[23–25] to no association.[26] However, in longitudinal studies, subjective cognitive impairments have been associated with higher rates of incident cognitive impairment and dementia.[22,27–29] Of note, multiple studies have shown that subjective cognitive impairments are common in individuals with late-life depression, with ranges falling from 50% to 70%.[30,31] Interestingly, one prospective study showed that tau-mediated degeneration, but not beta-amyloid (Aβ) deposition, was significantly higher in patients with MCI compared with SCI.[32] At this time, although there seems to be compelling evidence of a relationship between SCI and depression, further research is needed to more fully understand the causal relationship between the two.

Mild Cognitive Impairment and Depression

MCI is characterized by cognitive complaints (per the patients, informants, or observed by a clinician), objective evidence of impairment, independence in functional abilities, and no impairment in social or occupational functioning.[33] The prevalence of depression in MCI varies widely, with population-based estimates ranging from 3.0% to 83.0%, with a median prevalence of 44.3%; alternatively, the prevalence of MCI in depression ranges from 30% to 50%.[34–36] For most individuals with late-life depression and comorbid cognitive impairment, the profile seems to be a dys-executive pattern[37] characterized by difficulties with working memory, set-shifting, planning, and response inhibition. This syndrome suggests that cerebrovascular disease affects white matter tracts in the fronto-striatal pathways, resulting in executive dysfunction and, potentially, the affective symptoms of depression. Additionally, studies have found that late-life depression is associated with a higher ischemic burden on structural MRI as well as impaired executive and memory functions.[38,39]

Dementia and Depression

Longitudinal studies have provided information on the cognitive trajectories of those with late-life depression. Potter and colleagues[40] found that baseline impairments in encoding and executive functioning in patients with depression seem to be risk factors for progression to dementia. However, this progression seems to be highly variable. Steffens and colleagues[41] found that in a large group of nondemented depressed older adults, at the 2-year follow-up approximately 25% had reverted back to normal cognitive functioning, 15% had progressed to dementia, and the remainder continued to display cognitive impairments without functional decline. Additional research has shown that although one would expect most individuals with late-life depression and MCI to progress to a vascular dementia, these vascular risk factors may simply serve to accelerate the AD process.[34,42]

BIOMARKERS
Apolipoprotein E, Beta-Amyloid, and Tau

Studies on various markers in neurodegenerative illnesses (ie, apolipoprotein E ε4 variant [APOE ε4], Aβ, and tau) and late-life depression have been variable. Regarding APOE ε4, there seems to be a significant relationship between depressive symptoms and APOE ε4 in regard to progression from MCI to dementia. Specifically, a longitudinal study showed that APOE ε4 carriers with depression were 4.4 times more likely to progress to AD compared with non-APOE ε4 carriers with depression.[43] Meanwhile, a cross-sectional study found no relationship between APOE ε4 status, depression, and cognition.[44] Further research on the relation between Aβ and APOE ε4 is mixed.[45–48] Finally, although the relationship between tau protein and late-life depression has not yet been clearly established, a longitudinal study indicated those with late-life depression and elevated cerebrospinal fluid total tau levels progressed differently from MCI to AD.[49,50]

Neurotrophins

Recent literature has indicated that individuals with late-life depression display a reduction of neurotrophins, including nerve growth factor, glial-derived neurotrophic factor, and brain-derived neurotrophic factor.[51–53] However, Arnold and colleagues[54] found that 2 neurotrophins specifically associated with neurogenesis, long-term potentiation, and response to ischemic injuries seemed to be increased in older adults with depressive symptoms: vascular endothelial growth factor and hepatocyte growth factor (reflecting possible compensatory responses).

Hippocampal-Pituitary-Adrenal Axis, Insulin Pathway, and Inflammation

There is limited evidence suggesting that the hippocampal-pituitary-adrenal (HPA) axis and inflammation play a role in late-life depression with comorbid cognitive deficits. Although chronic distress has been associated with disruption in the HPA axis, research on this relationship with comorbid cognitive impairments has been variable.[54,55] Interestingly, literature has provided compelling evidence of hippocampal atrophy in individuals with severe depression and positive inflammation biomarkers.[56]

NEUROIMAGING AND ELECTROPHYSIOLOGY
Structural MRI

With structural MRI, changes in both white and gray matter have been associated with late-life depression and comorbid cognitive impairment compared with nondepressed older adults. In support of the vascular hypothesis, suggesting that cerebrovascular disease is a major contributor to late-life depression, longitudinal MRI studies have shown a correlation between the severity of depression and white matter ischemic changes.[57,58] Similarly, these white matter lesions, especially when concentrated in anterior periventricular regions, have been associated with comorbid executive dysfunction.

Gray matter changes seen in late-life depression may be part of the prodrome to AD. Hippocampal atrophy, a well-known feature of AD, has also been shown to be associated with a higher severity of emotional distress in nondemented individuals.[59] For individuals with MCI, depression was associated with reduced thickness of the entorhinal cortex, anterior cingulate cortex, and bilateral dorsomedial and ventromedial prefrontal cortices.[60–62]

Functional MRI

The connectome (how the brain functions as a system of multiple connected networks) and how pathophysiologic processes can disrupt the connectome are now major areas of research. Recent functional MRI studies suggest that structural lesions associated with late-life depression can also lead to the disruption of networks associated with the clinical features in late-life depression (eg, apathy and executive dysfunction). In one study, the cognitive control network and corticostriatal networks were shown to be linked to cognitive dysfunction (ie, executive impairments) in late-life depression.[63]

PET Imaging and Florbetapir Imaging

PET imaging studies provide conflicting information. Specifically, one study found that some patients with late-life depression and MCI showed a Pittsburgh compound B imaging pattern suggestive of AD,[64] whereas another did not replicate this relationship.[65] Research with an amyloid and neurofibrillary tangle binding agent (FDDNP) for individuals with MCI and depression found variable temporal and parietal lobe binding.[66,67] This finding was further confirmed by research coming from the Alzheimer's Disease Neuroimaging Initiative showing that lifelong depressive symptoms reliably predicted Aβ accumulation in patients with MCI.[68] These findings suggest that larger studies are needed to understand the complex PET imaging relationship between depression and cognitive impairment.

Electrophysiology Markers

Using electroencephalogram (EEG) technology, individuals with late-life depression have shown more slow-wave activity and prolonged $P300_a$ latencies, indicating decreased cerebral arousal and information processing.[69] Additional researching using a complex response inhibition task showed decreased event potential localized to the anterior cingulate cortex in depressed older adults.[70] Although not diagnostic, these EEG findings may help shed light on the cognitive deficits often reported by individuals with late-life depression.

PSYCHOTHERAPIES

Several evidence-based psychotherapies have been shown to be effective in the treatment of late-life depression, even in those with associated cognitive impairments. Psychotherapy should always be considered for individuals with MCI and early AD, especially, as older adults typically only show an adequate response in approximately 30% after a trial of a first-line antidepressant.[71]

Cognitive Behavioral Therapy

Cognitive-behavioral therapy (CBT) has become one of the more common treatments for a wide-range of disorders, including depression, posttraumatic stress disorder, anxiety, insomnia, and so forth. It is based on the assumption that maladaptive patterns of thought and behavior contribute to the development of emotional distress, such as depression. CBT focuses on breaking the links between dysfunctional cognitions, emotions, and behaviors. One recent meta-analysis[72] found that CBT and problem-solving therapy (PST) were more effective than other therapies in treating late-life depression. Furthermore, research has shown CBT to be effective even when applied to individuals with MCI.[73]

Interpersonal Therapy

Interpersonal therapy (IPT) concludes that the development of depressive symptoms is influenced by the relationships between patients and their significant others. For treatment, it combines techniques from supportive and psychodynamic therapies, focusing on interactions between the therapists and the patients, with the goal of generalizing positive interactions toward the patients' significant others. IPT has been shown to be effective in the treatment of treatment-resistant depression for younger to middle-aged adults,[74] although there are fewer studies in older adults. One study[75] showed that IPT, when modified to include patients' caregivers, was effective in reducing depressive symptoms in cognitively impaired individuals.

Problem-Solving Therapy

PST focuses treatment on everyday problems, with the goal of improving coping skills to prevent distress. The therapists work with the patients to identify problems, develop a set of possible solutions, decide on one of these solutions, and then implement the solution (assessing its success). Two meta-analyses[76,77] have shown that PST effectively treats late-life depression. Furthermore, these findings are supported by another meta-analysis indicating PST was more effective than several other psychotherapies.[72] In a multisite clinical trial of older adults with depression and executive dysfunction, problem-solving was shown to be more effective than supportive therapy in reducing depressive symptoms (persisting long after the 12 weeks of treatment).[78] Furthermore, late-life depression seems responsive to modified PSTs, including primary care–based PST, problem adaptation therapy, and home-bound PST for individual with cognitive impairments.[79–81]

Reminiscence and Life Review

Based on Erikson's last stage of life span development focused on "meaning making," reminiscence and life review therapies were designed to treat psychological disorders in older adults. The life review is a systematic process structured around life themes, such as one's childhood, parenthood, work productivity, and so forth. For treatment, the therapists work with the patients to recall memories with the goal of focusing on positive life events and enhancing well-being. The life review process then focuses on developing a narrative of the person's life, evaluating events and reframing and integrating them. There are 3 meta-analyses that have shown reminiscence and life review therapies to be effective in treating late-life depression[72,82,83]; however, these data were complicated by the variations in how these therapies are applied.

HOLISTIC AND OTHER NONTRADITIONAL APPROACHES

Because of a variety of reasons, for many older adults, holistic and other nontraditional approaches for treatment of depression may be more acceptable than psychopharmacologic and psychotherapeutic approaches. First, as nontraditional treatments (eg, physical activity, art therapy, meditation, and so forth) have been used by many for non–mental health reasons, older adults may be more open to their use, especially if they have no history of psychiatric treatment. Second, older adults may find it easier to speak with their physicians about their physical symptoms than their emotional or cognitive complaints. Therefore, offering holistic and nontraditional treatments, which may benefit both physical and mental health, may be more acceptable. Third, as the mental health community has grown in the integration and study of nontraditional treatments, the authors have found that, although not easy to study, these approaches may offer unique benefits for the treatment of late-life depression.[84]

Physical Activity and Cognitive Training

Physical exercise has been shown to have a significant impact on both late-life depression and cognition. A systematic review by Mura and Carta[85] showed that most of the included studies showed reductions in depressive symptoms (with no other interventions used). Multiple studies have shown that exercise alone is equally effective, if not a powerful addition, to antidepressant medications.[86–88] Moreover, exercise has the potential to improve cognitive functioning in older adults as well. Particularly, executive functions, for example, planning, working memory, problem-solving, and so forth, seem to have robust benefits from aerobic exercise.[89]

There also seems to be some evidence that cognitive training may have some cognitive benefits in depressed older adults.[90,91] However, further research needs to be done to examine generalization from these effects to daily functioning.

Technological Interventions

Recent advances have allowed technological approaches to be combined with traditional treatments of mental health issues. Internet-based psychotherapies[92] and exergaming[93] can function independently or be further augmented with the use of mobile applications.[94] However, there is not yet compelling evidence for the effectiveness of these approaches with older adults.

Religion and Spirituality

With the increased importance of cultural competency in mental health research, the role of religious and spirituality practices has gained recognition for the treatment of late-life depression. For example, studies on the use of yoga and meditation have shown significant reductions in depressive symptoms in older adults.[95,96] However, the effects these practices have on cognition are not yet well known. Finally, research on the use of tai chi with older adults suggests improvements in depressive symptoms, physical functioning, and cognitive functioning as well as reductions in inflammatory C-reactive protein.[97,98]

Music, Art, and Dance Therapy

Various art therapies have been shown to have positive effects on both mood and cognition. Specifically, music therapy may improve depression and cognitive symptoms in older adults[99,100] and dance therapy has shown a significant effect on mood.[101,102]

Ketamine

Recent literature has indicated that ketamine, typically used as an intravenous anesthetic, has been shown to have rapid antidepressant efficacy in individuals with refractory major depressive disorder (MDD).[103] Moreover, initial studies have not shown there to be lasting neurocognitive deficits secondary to ketamine treatment 1 week after administration, although there is an initial slowing in processing speed.[104]

PHARMACOLOGIC APPROACHES
Antidepressants

Most of the recent literature on depression and cognition has focused on selective serotonin reuptake inhibitors (SSRIs) and selective serotonin-norepinephrine reuptake inhibitors (SNRIs). The results on SSRIs have been variable, depending largely on the medication being studied. Specifically, sertraline was indicated to improve episodic memory and executive functions,[9] whereas citalopram was shown to cause difficulties in response inhibition, verbal learning, and processing speed.[105,106] Alternatively, there seems to be more compelling evidence of cognitive benefits from SNRIs.[107,108] Alternatively, antidepressants with anticholinergic effects (ie, many tricyclic antidepressants) likely have detrimental effects on cognition.[109]

Cholinesterase Inhibitors and N-Methyl-D-Aspartate Antagonists

Research on the use of cholinesterase inhibitors for late-life depression and comorbid MCI are limited, with conflicting findings in terms of cognitive and mood outcomes. Interestingly, research on donepezil has shown varying results, from positive effects on depression[110,111] to no positive effects.[112] Memantine, an N-methyl-D-aspartate antagonist, has not been shown to have any efficacy as a treatment of comorbid MDD.[113–115]

BRAIN STIMULATION THERAPIES
Electroconvulsive Therapy

Although initially developed for the treatment of psychotic symptoms, ECT has been shown to be effective in the treatment of severe, treatment-resistant depression.[116] Although not fully understood, ECT is thought to release multiple neurotransmitters, including glutamate, noradrenalin, dopamine, and serotonin.[117,118] However, post-ECT cognitive adverse effects have been found. These effects tend to be time limited and include disorientation after each ECT session and both anterograde and retrograde amnesia, which can persist for 1 to 6 months after the last session.[117,119] More subtle cognitive deficits have also been shown to be time limited and include decreases in processing speed, working memory, learning and memory, and executive functions.[120,121]

Other Brain-Stimulation Therapies

Rather than using an electrical current, transcranial magnetic stimulation (TMS) uses an electromagnet to stimulate brain regions. In one study, patients receiving repetitive TMS showed improvement in depressive symptoms, functioning, and cognitive performances.[122–124] Although not yet used to study late-life depression with comorbid depression, this intervention seems to be a promising area of future research.

Although deep brain stimulation (DBS) has been shown to be associated with successful outcomes for treatment-resistant depression, responses differ among studies, with 6-month success rates ranging from 41% to 66%.[125–128] Several DBS targets have been studied, including the subgenual cingulate region, subcallosal tracts, nucleus accumbens, ventral striatum, inferior thalamic peduncle, and habenula. At this time, there is not compelling evidence for cognitive benefits of DBS for patients with late-life depression and comorbid cognitive impairment.

SUMMARY

Although the understanding of the relationship between depression and cognition has grown significantly over the past several years, researchers continue to uncover more details regarding the complex interplay between these two factors. There have been several promising developments recently, especially with advances in neuroimaging and biomarker research. Additionally, although several therapeutic modalities have been researched for the treatment of late-life depression, many of them have been limited by factors, including providers' experience and/or treatment availability. Given the current literature, optimal assessment and treatment of older adults with depression should include multiple modalities, such as neuroimaging, genotyping, and risk factor burden calculations, to better understand the patients' prognosis and potential treatment response. Future research should then focus on more individualized treatments, pharmacologic and psychotherapeutic, for late-life depression in order to more effectively treat both cognitive and affective symptoms.

ACKNOWLEDGMENTS

The authors thank Dr Fred Unverzagt for his irreplaceable expertise in this field and his valuable contributions to this body of work.

REFERENCES

1. Eden J, LeM, Maslow K, et al, editors. The mental health and substance use workforce for older adults: in whose hands? Washington, DC: Natl. Acad. Press; 2012.

2. Byers AL, Yaffe K. Depression and risk of developing dementia. Nat Rev Neurol 2011;7:323–31.

3. Steenland K, Karnes C, Seals R, et al. Late-life depression as a risk factor for mild cognitive impairment or Alzheimer's disease in 30 US Alzheimer's disease centers. J Alzheimers Dis 2012;31:265–75.

4. Blazer D. Depression in late life: review and commentary. J Gerontol A Biol Sci Med Sci 2003;58(3):249–65.

5. Karyotaki E, Smit Y, Holdt Henningsen K, et al. Combining pharmacotherapy and psychotherapy or monotherapy for major depression? A meta-analysis on the long-term effects. J Affect Disord 2016;194:144–52.

6. Islam MM, Iqbal U, Walther B, et al. Benzodiazepine use and rick of dementia in the elderly population: a systematic review and meta-analysis. Neuroepidemiology 2016;47(3–4):181–91.

7. Blank K. Older adults & substance use: new data highlight concerns. SAMHSA News, Jan–Feb. 2009. Available at: http://www.samhsa.gov/. Accessed June 12, 2017.

8. Apostolova LG, Di LJ, Duffy EL, et al. Risk factors for behavioral abnormalities in mild cognitive impairment and mild Alzheimer's disease. Dement Geriatr Cogn Disord 2014;37:315–26.

9. Barch DM, D'Angelo G, Pieper C, et al. Cognitive improvement following treatment in late-life depression: relationship to vascular risk and age of onset. Am J Geriatr Psychiatry 2012;20:682–90.

10. Sheline YI, Pieper CF, Wlesh-Bohmer K, et al. Support for the vascular depression hypothesis in late-life depression: results of a 2-site, prospective, antidepressant treatment trial. Arch Gen Psychiatry 2010;67(3):277–85.

11. Agganis BT, Weiner DE, Giang LM, et al. Depression and cognitive function in maintenance hemodialysis patients. Am J Kidney Dis 2010;56:704–12.

12. Elias MF, Dore GA, Davey A. Kidney disease and cognitive function. Contrib Nephrol 2013;179:42–57.

13. Doyle T, Palmer S, Johnson J, et al. Association of anxiety and depression with pulmonary-specific symptoms in chronic obstructive pulmonary disease. Int J Psychiatry Med 2013;45:189–202.

14. Bratek A, Zawada K, Beil-Gawelczyk J, et al. Depressiveness, symptoms of anxiety and cognitive dysfunctions in patients with asthma and chronic obstructive pulmonary disease (COPD): possible associations with inflammation markers: a pilot study. J Neural Trans (Vienna) 2015;122:S83–91.

15. Am Found Suicide Prev. Facts and figures. New York: Am. Found. Suicide Prev; 2012. Available at. https://www.afsp.org/understanding-suicide/facts-and-figures.

16. Conwell Y, Van Orden K, Caine ED. Suicide in older adults. Psychiatr Clin N Am 2011;34:451–68.

17. Szanto K, Dombrovski AY, Sahakian BJ, et al. Social emotion recognition, social functioning, and attempted suicide in late-life depression. Am J Geriatr Psychiatry 2012;20:257–65.

18. Chan SS, Lyness JM, Conwell Y. Do cerebrovascular risk factors confer risk for suicide in later life? A case-control study. Am J Geriatr Psychiatry 2007;15:541–4.

19. Kurella M, Kimmel PL, Young BS, et al. Suicide in the United States end-stage renal disease program. J Am Soc Nephrol 2005;16:774–81.

20. Blazer DG, Wallace RB. Cognitive aging: what every geriatric psychiatrist should know. J Geriatr Psychiatry 2016;24:776–81.

21. Harada CN, Natelson Love MC, Triebel KL. Normal cognitive aging. Clin Geriatr Med 2013;29(4):737–52.

22. Hill NL, Mogle J, Wion R, et al. Subjective cognitive impairment and affective symptoms: a systematic review. J Gerontologist 2016;56(6):e109–27.

23. Amariglio RE, Townsend MK, Grodstein F, et al. Specific subjective memory complaints in older persons may indicate poor cognitive function. J Am Geriatr Soc 2011;59(9):1612–7.
24. Jonker C, Launer LJ, Hooijer C, et al. Memory complaints and memory impairment in older individuals. J Am Geriatr Soc 1996;44(1):44–9.
25. Montejo Carrasco P, Montenegro-Pena M, Lopez-Higes R, et al. Subjective memory complaints in healthy older adults: fewer complaints associated with depression and perceived health, more complaints also associated with lower memory performance. Arch Gerontol Geriat 2017;70:28–37.
26. Minett TS, Da Silva RV, Ortiz KZ, et al. Subjective memory complaints in an elderly sample: a cross sectional study. Int J Geriatr Psychiatry 2008;23(1): 49–54.
27. Dufouil C, Fuhrer R, Alperovitch A. Subjective cognitive complaints and cognitive decline: consequence or predictor? The epidemiology of vascular aging study. J Am Geriatr Soc 2005;53(4):616–21.
28. Waldorff FB, Siersma V, Vogel A, et al. Subjective memory complaints in general practice predicts future dementia: a 4-year follow-up study. Int J Geriatr Psychiatry 2012;27(11):1180–8.
29. Wang S, Blazer DG. Depression and cognition in the elderly. Annu Rev Clin Psychol 2015;11:331–60.
30. Bartley M, Bokde AL, Ewers M, et al. Subjective memory complaints in community dwelling healthy older people: the influence of brain and psychopathology. Int. J Geriatr Psychiatry 2012;27(8):836–43.
31. Chu CS, Sun IW, Begum A, et al. The association between subjective memory complaint and objective cognitive function in older people with previous major depression. PLoS One 2017;12(3):e0173027.
32. Wolfsgruber S, Polcher A, Koppara A, et al. Cerebrospinal fluid biomarkers and clinical progression in patients with subjective cognitive decline and mild cognitive impairment. J Alzheimers Dis 2017;58(3):939–50.
33. Langa KM, Levine DA. The diagnosis and management of mild cognitive impairment: a clinical review. JAMA 2014;312(23):2551–61.
34. Bhalla RK, Butters MA, Becker JT, et al. Patterns of mild cognitive impairment after treatment of depression in the elderly. Am J Geriatr Psychiatry 2009;17: 308–16.
35. Reinlieb M, Ercoli LM, Siddarth P, et al. The patterns of cognitive and functional impairment in amnestic and non-amnestic mild cognitive impairment in geriatric depression. Am J Geriatr Psychiatry 2014;22:1487–95.
36. Yeh YC, Tsang HY, Lin PY, et al. Subtypes of mild cognitive impairment among the elderly with major depressive disorder in remission. Am J Geriatr Psychiatry 2011;19:923–31.
37. Morimoto SS, Alexopoulos GS. Cognitive deficits in geriatric depression: clinical correlates and implications for current and future treatment. Psychiatr Clin N Am 2013;36:517–31.
38. Mackin RS, Nelson JC, Delucchi KL, et al. Association of age at depression onset with cognitive functioning in individuals with late-life depression and executive dysfunction. Am J Geriatr Psychiatry 2014;22:1633–41.
39. Salloway S, Malloy P, Kohn R, et al. MRI and neuropsychological differences in early- and late-life-onset geriatric depression. Neurology 1996;46:1567–74.
40. Potter GG, Wagner HR, Burke JR, et al. Neuropsychological predictors of dementia in late-life major depressive disorder. Am J Geriatr Psychiatry 2013;21: 297–306.

41. Steffens DC, McQuoid DR, Potter GG. Outcomes of older cognitively impaired individuals with current and past depression in the NCODE study. J Geriatr Psychiatry Neurol 2009;22:52–61.

42. Koenig AM, Bhalla RK, Meryl AB. Cognitive functioning and late-life depression. J Int Neuropsychol Soc 2014;20:1–7.

43. Irie F, Masaki KH, Petrovitch H, et al. Apolipoprotein E epsilon4 allele genotype and the effect of depressive symptoms on the risk of dementia in men: the Honolulu-Asia aging study. Arch Gen Psychiatry 2008;65:906–12.

44. Bogner HR, Richie MB, de Vries HF, et al. Depression, cognition, and apolipoprotein E genotype: latent class approach to identifying subtype. Am Geriatr Psychiatry 2009;17:344–52.

45. Blasko I, Kemmler G, Jungwirth S, et al. Plasma amyloid beta-42 independently predicts both late-onset depression and Alzheimer disease. Am J Geriatr Psychiatry 2010;18:973–82.

46. Metti AL, Cauley JA, Newman AB, et al. Plasma beta amyloid level and depression in older adults. J Gerontol A Biol Sci Med Sci 2013;68:74–9.

47. Sun X, Chiu CC, Liebson E, et al. Depression and plasma amyloid beta peptides in the elderly with and without the apolipoprotein E4 allele. Alzheimer Dis Assoc Disord 2009;23:238–44.

48. Szanto K, Clark L, Hallquist M, et al. The cost of social punishment and high-lethality suicide attempts in the second half of life. Psychol Aging 2014;29: 84–94.

49. Schonknecht P, Pantel J, Kaiser E, et al. Increased tau protein differentiates mild cognitive impairment from geriatric depression and predicts conversion to dementia. Neurosci Lett 2007;416:39–42.

50. Scogin F, Fairchild JK, Yon A, et al. Cognitive bibliotherapy and memory training for older adults with depressive symptoms. Aging Ment Health 2014;18:554–60.

51. Diniz BS, Teixeira AL, Machado-Vieira R, et al. Reduced serum nerve growth factor in patients with late-life depression. Am J Geriatr Psychiatry 2013;21: 493–6.

52. Diniz BS, Teixeira AL, Miranda AS, et al. Circulating glial-derived neurotrophic factor is reduced in late-life depression. J Psychiatr Res 2012;46:135–9.

53. Erickson KI, Miller DL, Roecklein KA. The aging hippocampus: interactions between exercise, depression, and BDNF. Neuroscientist 2012;18:82–97.

54. Arnold SE, Xie SX, Leung YY, et al. Plasma biomarkers of depressive symptoms in older adults. Transl Psychiatry 2012;3(2):e65.

55. Kohler S, Thomas AJ, Lloyd A, et al. White matter hyperintensities, cortisol levels, brain atrophy and continuing cognitive deficits in late-life depression. Br J Psychiatry 2010;196:143–9.

56. Sapolsky RM. Glucocorticoids and hippocampal atrophy in neuropsychiatric disorders. Arch Gen Psychiatry 2000;57:925–35.

57. Krishnan KR, Taylor WD, McQuoid DR, et al. Clinical characteristics of magnetic resonance imaging–defined subcortical ischemic depression. Biol Psychiatry 2004;55:390–7.

58. Taylor WD, Aizenstein HJ, Alexopoulos GS. The vascular depression hypothesis: mechanisms linking vascular disease with depression. Mol Psychiatry 2013;18: 963–74.

59. Taylor WD, McQuoid DR, Payne ME, et al. Hippocampus atrophy and the longitudinal course of late-life depression. Am J Geriatr Psychiatry 2014;22:1504–12.

60. Lebedeva AK, Westman E, Borza T, et al. MRI-based classification models in prediction of mild cognitive impairment and dementia in late-life depression. Front Aging Neurosci 2017;2:9–13.

61. Xie C, Li W, Chen G, et al. The co-existence of geriatric depression and amnestic mild cognitive impairment detrimentally affect gray matter volumes: voxel-based morphometry study. Behav Brain Res 2012;235:244–50.

62. Zahodne LB, Gongvatana A, Cohen RA, et al. Are apathy and depression independently associated with longitudinal trajectories of cortical atrophy in mild cognitive impairment? Am J Geriatr Psychiatry 2013;21:1098–106.

63. Tadayonnejad R, Ajilore O. Brain network dysfunction in late-life depression: a literature review. J Geriatr Psychiatry Neurol 2014;27:5–12.

64. Butters MA, Klunk WE, Mathis CA, et al. Imaging Alzheimer pathology in late-life depression with PET and Pittsburgh compound-B. Alzheimer Dis Assoc Disord 2008;22:261–8.

65. Madsen K, Hasselbalch BJ, Frederiksen KS, et al. Lack of association between prior depressive episodes and cerebral [11C]PiB binding. Neurobiol Aging 2012;33:2334–42.

66. Kumar A, Kepe V, Barrio JR, et al. Protein binding in patients with late-life depression. Arch Gen Psychiatry 2011;68:1143–50.

67. Lavretsky H, Siddarth P, Kepe V, et al. Depression and anxiety symptoms are associated with cerebral FDDNP-PET binding in middle-aged and older nondemented adults. Am J Geriatr Psychiatry 2009;17:493–502.

68. Chung JK, Plitman E, Nakajima S, et al. Lifetime history of depression predicts increased amyloid-B accumulation in patients with mild cognitive impairment. J Alzheimers Dis 2015;45(3):907–19.

69. Kohler S, Ashton CH, Marsh R, et al. Electrophysiological changes in late life depression and their relation to structural brain changes. Int Psychogeriatr 2011;23:141–8.

70. Katza R, De Sanctisa P, Mahoneya JR, et al. Cognitive control in late-life depression: response inhibition deficits and dysfunction of the anterior cingulate cortex. Am J Geriatr Psychiatry 2010;18:1017–25.

71. Lenze EJ, Sheffrin M, Driscoll HC, et al. Incomplete response in late-life depression: getting to remission. Dialogues Clin Neurosci 2008;10:419–30.

72. Cuijpers P, Karyotaki E, Pot AM, et al. Managing depression in older age: psychological interventions. Maturitas 2014;79(2):160–9.

73. Joosten-Weyn Banningh LW, Kessels RP, Olde Rikkert MG, et al. A cognitive behavioural group therapy for patients diagnosed with mild cognitive impairment and their significant others: feasibility and preliminary results. Clin Rehabil 2008;22:731–40.

74. Hollon SD, Ponniah K. A review of empirically supported psychological therapies for mood disorders in adults. Depress Anxiety 2010;27(10):891–932.

75. Miller MD, Reynolds CF 3rd. Expanding the usefulness of interpersonal psychotherapy (IPT) for depressed elders with co-morbid cognitive impairment. Int J Geriatr Psychiatry 2007;22:101–5.

76. Bell AC, D'Zurilla TJ. Problem-solving therapy for depression: a meta-analysis. Clin Psychol Rev 2009;29(4):348–53.

77. Malouff JM, Thorsteinsson EB, Schutte NS. The efficacy of problem solving therapy in reducing mental and physical health problems: a meta-analysis. Clin Psychol Rev 2007;27(1):46–57.

78. Alexopoulos GS, Raue PJ, Kiosse sDN, et al. Problem-solving therapy and supportive therapy in older adults with major depression and executive dysfunction: effect on disability. Arch Gen Psychiatry 2011;68:33–41.

79. Arean P, Hegel M, Vannoy S, et al. Effectiveness of problem-solving therapy for older, primary care patients with depression: results from the IMPACT project. Gerontologist 2008;48:311–23.

80. Arean PA, Raue P, Mackin RS, et al. Problem-solving therapy and supportive therapy in older adults with major depression and executive dysfunction. Am J Psychiatry 2010;167:1391–8.

81. Kiosses DN, Arean PA, Teri L, et al. Home-delivered problem adaptation therapy (PATH) for depressed, cognitively impaired, disabled elders: a preliminary study. Am J Geriatr Psychiatry 2010;18:988–98.

82. Bohlmeijer E, Smit F, Cuijpers P. Effects of reminiscence and life review on late-life depression: a meta-analysis. Int J Geriatr Psychiatry 2003;18(12):1088–94.

83. Pinquart M, Forstmeijer S. Effects of reminiscence interventions on psychosocial outcomes: a meta-analysis. Aging Ment Health 2012;16(5):541–58.

84. Ventegodt S, Merrick J. Meta-analysis of positive effects, side effects and adverse events of holistic mind-body medicine (clinical holistic medicine): experience from Denmark, Sweden, United Kingdom and Germany. Int J Adolesc Med Health 2009;21(4):441–56.

85. Mura G, Carta MG. Physical activity in depressed elderly: a systematic review. Clin Pract Epidemiol Ment Health 2013;9:125–35.

86. Blumenthal JA, Babyak MA, Moore KA, et al. Effects of exercise training on older patients with major depression. Arch Intern Med 1999;159(19):2349–56.

87. Bogner HR, Bruce ML, Reynolds CF 3rd, et al. The effects of memory, attention, and executive dysfunction on outcomes of depression in a primary care intervention trial: the PROSPECT study. Int J Geriatr Psychiatry 2007;22:922–9.

88. Mather AS, Rodriguez C, Guthrie MF, et al. Effects of exercise on depressive symptoms in older adults with poorly responsive depressive disorder: randomised controlled trial. Br J Psychiatry 2002;180:411–5.

89. Northey JM, Cherbuin N, Pumpa KL, et al. Exercise interventions for cognitive function in adults older than 50: a systematic review with meta-analysis. Br J Sports Med 2017. [Epub ahead of print].

90. Mowszowski L, Hermens DF, Diamond K, et al. Cognitive training enhances pre-attentive neurophysiological responses in older adults "at risk" of dementia. J Alzheimers Dis 2014;41(4):1095–108.

91. Naismith SL, Diamond K, Carter PE, et al. Enhancing memory in late-life depression: the effects of a combined psychoeducation and cognitive training program. Am J Geriatr Psychiatry 2011;19:240–8.

92. Donker T, Batterham PJ, Warmerdam L, et al. Predictors and moderators of response to Internet-delivered interpersonal psychotherapy and cognitive behavior therapy for depression. J Affect Disord 2013;151:343–51.

93. Rosenberg D, Depp CA, Vahia IV, et al. Exergames for subsyndromal depression in older adults: a pilot study of a novel intervention. Am J Geriatr Psychiatry 2010;18:221–6.

94. Donker T, Petrie K, Proudfoot J, et al. Smartphones for smarter delivery of mental health programs: a systematic review. J Med Internet Res 2013;15:e247.

95. Nash JD, Newberg A. Toward a unifying taxonomy and definition for meditation. Front Psychol 2013;4:806.

96. Patel NK, Newstead AH, Ferrer RL. The effects of yoga on physical functioning and health related quality of life in older adults: a systematic review and meta-analysis. J Altern Complement Med 2012;18:902–17.

97. Lavretsky H, Alstein LL, Olmstead RE, et al. Complementary use of tai chi chih augments escitalopram treatment of geriatric depression: a randomized controlled trial. Am J Geriatr Psychiatry 2011;19:839–50.

98. Rogers CE, Larkey LK, Keller C. A review of clinical trials of tai chi and qigong in older adults. West J Nurs Res 2009;31:245–79.

99. Cross K, Flores R, Butterfield J, et al. The effect of passive listening versus active observation of music and dance performances on memory recognition and mild to moderate depression in cognitively impaired older adults. Psychol Rep 2012;111:413–23.

100. Hars M, Herrmann FR, Gold G, et al. Effect of music-based multitask training on cognition and mood in older adults. Age Ageing 2014;43:196–200.

101. McCaffrey R, Liehr P, Gregersen T, et al. Garden walking and art therapy for depression in older adults: a pilot study. Res Gerontol Nurs 2011;4:237–42.

102. Murrock CJ, Graor CH. The effects of dance on depression, physical function, and disability in underserved adults. J Aging Phys Act 2014;22(3):380–5.

103. Pehrson AL, Sanchez C. Serotonergic modulation of glutamate neurotransmission as a strategy for treating depression and cognitive dysfunction. CNS Spectr 2014;19:121–33.

104. Murrough JW, Burdick KE, Levitch CF, et al. Neurocognitive effects of ketamine and association with antidepressant response in individuals with treatment-resistant depression: a randomized controlled trial. Neuropsychopharmacology 2015;40(5):1084–90.

105. Pimontel MA, Culang-Reinlieb ME, Morimoto SS, et al. Executive dysfunction and treatment response in late-life depression. Int J Geriatr Psychiatry 2012; 27:893–9.

106. Sneed JR, Culang ME, Keilp JG, et al. Antidepressant medication and executive dysfunction: a deleterious interaction in late-life depression. Am J Geriatr Psychiatry 2010;18:128–35.

107. Raskin J, Wiltse CG, Siegal A, et al. Efficacy of duloxetine on cognition, depression, and pain in elderly patients with major depressive disorder: an 8-week, double-blind, placebo-controlled trial. Am J Psychiatry 2007;164:900–9.

108. Wesnes K, Bose A, Gommoll C, Chen C. Effects of levomilnacipran SR on measures of attention in a phase 3 trial of major depressive disorder (MDD). Presented at NCDEU 53rdMeet., Am. Soc. Clin. Psychopharmacol., Hollywood, CA, May 28-31, 2013.

109. Khawam EA, Laurencic G, Malone DA. Side effects of antidepressants: an overview. Clevel Clin J Med 2006;73:351–3, 356–61.

110. Pelton GH, Harper OL, Tabert MH, et al. Randomized double-blind placebo-controlled donepezil augmentation in antidepressant-treated elderly patients with depression and cognitive impairment: a pilot study. Int J Geriatr Psychiatry 2008;23:670–6.

111. Reynolds CF 3rd, Butters MA, Lopez O, et al. Maintenance treatment of depression in old age: a randomized, double-blind, placebo-controlled evaluation of the efficacy and safety of donepezil combined with antidepressant pharmacotherapy. Arch Gen Psychiatry 2011;68:51–60.

112. Holtzheimer PE, Meeks TW, Kelley ME, et al. A double blind, placebo-controlled pilot study of galantamine augmentation of antidepressant treatment in older adults with major depression. Int J Geriatr Psychiatry 2008;23:625–31.

113. Lenze EJ, Skidmore ER, Begley AE, et al. Memantine for late-life depression and apathy after a disabling medical event: a 12-week, double-blind placebo-controlled pilot study. Int J Geriatr Psychiatry 2012;27:974–80.

114. Smith EG, Deligiannidis KM, Ulbricht CM, et al. Antidepressant augmentation using the N-methyl-D-aspartate antagonist memantine: a randomized, double-blind, placebo-controlled trial. J Clin Psychiatry 2013;74:966–73.

115. Zarate CA Jr, Singh JB, Quiroz JA, et al. A double-blind, placebo-controlled study of memantine in the treatment of major depression. Am J Psychiatry 2006;163:153–5.

116. Sackheim HA, Prudic J, Fuller R, et al. The cognitive effects of electroconvulsive therapy in community settings. Neuropsychopharmacology 2007;32:244–54.

117. Lisanby SH. Electroconvulsive therapy for depression. New Engl J Med 2007;357:1939–45.

118. Wahlund B, van Rosen D. ECT of major depressed patients in relation to biological and clinical variables: a brief overview. Neuropsychopharmacology 2003;28(Suppl 1):S21–6.

119. McClintock SM, Choi J, Deng ZD, et al. Multifactorial determinants of the neurocognitive effects of electroconvulsive therapy. J ECT 2014;30:165–76.

120. Semkovska M, McLoughlin DM. Objective cognitive performance associated with electroconvulsive therapy for depression: a systematic review and meta-analysis. Biol Psychiatry 2010;68:568–77.

121. Sheline YI, Barch DM, Garcia K, et al. Cognitive function in late life depression: relationships to depression severity, cerebrovascular risk factors and processing speed. Biol Psychiatry 2006;60:58–65.

122. Ahmed MA, Darwish ES, Khedr EM, et al. Effects of low versus high frequencies of repetitive transcranial magnetic stimulation on cognitive function and cortical excitability in Alzheimer's dementia. J Neurol 2012;259:83–92.

123. Alexopoulos GS, Hoptman MJ, Kanellopoulos D, et al. Functional connectivity in the cognitive control network and the default mode network in late-life depression. J Affect Disord 2012;139:56–65.

124. Alexopoulos GS, Murphy CF, Gunning-Dixon FM, et al. Microstructural white matter abnormalities and remission of geriatric depression. Am J Psychiatry 2008;165:238–44.

125. Drevets WC, Price JL, Furey ML. Brain structural and functional abnormalities in mood disorders: implications for neurocircuitry models of depression. Brain Struct Funct 2008;213(1–2):93–118.

126. Dubois B, Litvan I. The FAB: a frontal assessment battery at bedside. Neurology 2000;55:1621–6.

127. Greicius MD, Flores BH, Menon V, et al. Resting-state functional connectivity in major depression: abnormally increased contributions from subgenual cingulate cortex and thalamus. Biol Psychiatry 2007;62(5):429–37.

128. Kennedy SH, Giacobbe P, Rizvi SJ, et al. Deep brain stimulation for treatment-resistant depression: follow-up after 3 to 6 years. Am J Psychiatry 2011;168(5):502–10.

Managing Behavioral and Psychological Symptoms of Dementia

Lauren B. Gerlach, DO[a],*, Helen C. Kales, MD[a,b]

KEYWORDS

- Dementia • Behavioral and psychological symptoms of dementia
- Nonpharmacologic treatment • Caregivers

KEY POINTS

- Behavioral disturbances are universally experienced by people with dementia and cause significant impairment in quality of life, health care outcomes, and caregiver burden.
- Antipsychotics are typically used to treat such behaviors, although evidence to support their use is modest and associated with harms, including increased mortality. There are currently no FDA-approved medications for treatment of behavioral disturbances in dementia.
- Nonpharmacologic interventions, better termed "ecobiopsychosocial," are recommended first line and should target patient with dementia factors, caregiver factors, and environmental factors.
- The DICE (Describe, Investigate, Create, Evaluate) approach can provide a structured approach to investigating and treating behavioral and psychotic symptoms of dementia (BPSD).
- Pharmacologic measures should be considered first line for three specific scenarios: major depressive disorder with or without suicidal ideation, psychosis causing harm or potential for harm, and aggression with risk to self or others.

INTRODUCTION

Alzheimer disease and related dementias are among the most costly and distressing medical conditions for patients and their caregivers. In 2016 it was estimated that there were 5.2 million Americans with Alzheimer disease, with that number projected to increase to 13.8 million by 2050.[1,2] Alzheimer disease is currently the sixth leading cause of death within the United States and has costs of more than $236 billion

Disclosure: The authors have nothing to disclose.
[a] Program for Positive Aging, Department of Psychiatry, University of Michigan, 4250 Plymouth Road, Ann Arbor, MI 48109, USA; [b] Center for Clinical Management Research, VA Ann Arbor Healthcare System, 2215 Fuller Road, Ann Arbor, MI 48105, USA
* Corresponding author.
E-mail address: glauren@med.umich.edu

Psychiatr Clin N Am 41 (2018) 127–139
https://doi.org/10.1016/j.psc.2017.10.010
0193-953X/18/© 2017 Elsevier Inc. All rights reserved.

annually.[1] Families and caregivers of patients with dementia are greatly affected because most individuals with dementia are cared for within their home by family and friends.[3,4]

Although dementia is often thought of as a disease of memory, neuropsychiatric (eg, behavioral and psychological symptoms) and social deficits are nearly universal across all types and stages of dementia.[5] The Cache County study found that over the course of dementia, 97% of individuals with dementia experience one or more behavioral disturbance.[6] These behavioral and psychological symptoms of dementia (BPSD) can often be the most challenging for caregivers and families.

BEHAVIORAL AND PSYCHOLOGICAL SYMPTOMS OF DEMENTIA

BPSD, also known neuropsychiatric symptoms, occurs in clusters or syndromes identified as depression, psychosis (delusions and hallucinations), agitation, aggression, apathy, sleep disturbances, and disinhibition (socially and sexually inappropriate behaviors) (**Table 1**).[7] Agitation is often a broad category and it is helpful to clarify the specific behaviors that are of concern. Agitation can include restlessness, pacing, arguing, disruptive vocalizations, and rejection of care (eg, bathing, dressing, grooming).[7] Aggression is typically defined as verbal insults, such as shouting, and physical aggression, such as hitting and biting others, and throwing objects. In addition, there are numerous behaviors (eg, arguing, repetitive questions, resistance to care) that do not fit neatly into any symptom category, but are nonetheless burdensome to caregivers.[8]

Although BPSD is seen throughout the course of dementia illness, symptoms may occur intermittently or fluctuate greatly in severity. These behaviors are found in all types of dementia; however, some symptom clusters are more common in specific types of dementia. For instance, psychosis and visual hallucinations are more typical features of Lewy body dementia. Additionally, symptoms such as disinhibition, apathy, and social inappropriateness are often seen within frontotemporal dementia.

Table 1 Types of behavioral and psychological symptoms of dementia	
Agitation	Walking aimlessly Pacing Trailing Restlessness Repetitive actions
Aggression	Aggressive resistance Physical aggression Verbal aggression
Apathy	Withdrawn Lack of interest Amotivation
Depression	Sad Tearful Hopeless Anxiety Guilt
Psychosis	Hallucinations Delusions Misidentifications
Disinhibition	Socially and sexually inappropriate behavior

Although memory impairment is the hallmark of dementia, BPSD often can create the most challenges for patients, their caregivers, and providers.[9] These behaviors can change the trajectory for patients and are associated with faster disease progression[10] and increased morbidity and mortality.[11] Behavioral disturbances can often trigger nursing home placement and hospitalization, resulting in increased hospital length of stay.[11,12] BPSD is also associated with poor caregiver outcomes including increased caregiver stress and depression and reduced caregiver employment.[13] Roughly one-third of total dementia care costs are attributed to management of BPSD, related to increased service utilization, care costs, and caregiver time.[14]

CAUSES OF BEHAVIORAL AND PSYCHOLOGICAL SYMPTOMS OF DEMENTIA

Many factors have been found to be associated with the development of BPSD. Underlying many of these behaviors, there are fundamental changes and neurodegeneration in the brain of persons with dementia in centers that control cognition and emotion. Breakdown in this brain circuitry caused by dementia can impact the ability of the person with dementia to interact with others and their environment.[15] This can often lead to increased vulnerability to stressors, which can occur at the patient level, with the caregiver, and in the environment manifesting as behavioral disturbances.[7] As dementia progresses and communication becomes more difficult, behaviors should be seen as communications and caregivers need to rely more on a combination of strategies to understand what needs are being communicated. **Fig. 1** shows a

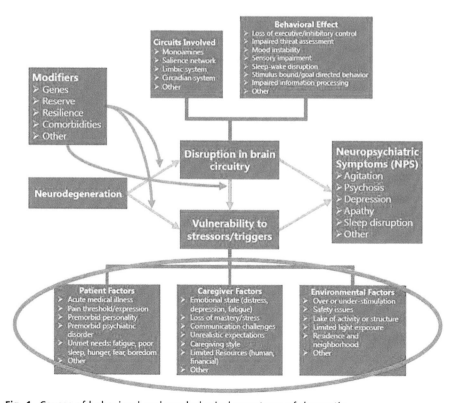

Fig. 1. Causes of behavioral and psychological symptoms of dementia.

conceptual model that details the myriad of causes of BPSD, which include person with dementia factors, caregiver factors, and environmental factors.

Person with Dementia Factors

Patient factors, such as an undiagnosed medical issue, can contribute to the development of behavioral disturbances. Medical issues, such as urinary tract infections, hypothyroidism, anemia, constipation, and pneumonia, are common culprits. In a study of community-dwelling older adults with dementia more than a third of patients were found to have undetected medical illnesses associated with behavioral disturbances.[16] Changes in central nervous system active medications, such as anticholinergic medications and opioids, and drug-drug interactions can lead to behavioral disturbances. Inadequate assessment and treatment of pain can lead to BPSD[17] with studies showing that empiric treatment of presumed pain can reduce agitation in residents of nursing homes with moderate to severe dementia.[18]

Additionally, premorbid personality traits, personality disorders, and psychiatric illness do not necessarily go away or diminish in the setting of a dementia diagnosis. Further disruptions in the neurocircuitry involved in the prefrontal cortex may worsen long-standing behavioral patterns caused by loss of "gating" or "top down inhibition."[15,19] Lastly, behaviors can be expressions of unmet needs or goals (physical, psychological, emotional, social).[20] Physical needs may include basic needs, such as thirst, hunger, or toileting. As patients with dementia lose the ability to communicate needs verbally, a trial and error approach by caregivers is needed to learn what the behavior might be representing.

Caregiver Factors

Dementia caregivers have higher levels of stress, lower levels of well-being, and worse physical health than noncaregivers and other caregivers.[21] Additionally caregivers of patients with BPSD have high rates of depression and anxiety.[1] Behavioral disturbances in patients are triggered or worsened when a caregiver is stressed or depressed.[22] Negative communication styles, such as anger, screaming, or an overly harsh tone, may also exacerbate behaviors. Caregivers may not understand what the patient with dementia can do at the particular stage of their illness and there can be a mismatch of expectations. Education to caregivers that a patient's behaviors are not volitional and that patients are not "doing this on purpose" are beneficial.

Environmental Factors

The environment is thought of interacting layers that comprise objects (items in the home), tasks (that compose activities of daily living), social groups, and culture (values and beliefs related to care in the home).[7] Individuals with dementia have difficulty processing and responding to stimuli in the environment. This lower stress threshold can lead to higher levels of frustration. Stress for patients with dementia may be increased by changes in routine or environment, overstimulation or understimulation in the environment, and demands that exceed functional ability.[23]

CURRENT TREATMENT

Given the complexity and multiple causes of BPSD, a "one-size fits all" treatment approach does not exist. It is important to understand the cause of symptoms, and knowing the underlying cause directs treatment. For instance, a urinary tract infection, pain, issues with caregivers, and psychosis are all approached differently.

Currently there are no Food and Drug Administration–approved medications for treatment of BPSD and all medications are considered off-label. Despite this, medications are often prescribed for treatment of BPSD and in real-world treatment settings patients with BPSD often receive an antipsychotic medication. Of all the drugs used for behaviors, antipsychotics do have the strongest evidence base, although the effect size is modest (0.13–0.16).[24,25] Any benefit must be balanced against risk of adverse events including mortality in this often medically frail population.[26–28] Based on mortality concerns, the FDA issued black box warnings for increased risk of mortality with use of atypical (2005) and typical (2008) antipsychotics in patients with dementia.[26,29] Causes of increased mortality are thought to be cardiovascular or cerebrovascular events and pneumonia.[28] Commonly used alternatives to antipsychotics, such as benzodiazepines and valproic acid, have even less evidence of positive risk/benefit ratios with no evidence for efficacy of these agents for treatment of BPSD other than sedation.[7]

NONPHARMACOLOGIC OR ECOBIOPSYCHOSOCIAL TREATMENT

Nonpharmacologic treatments for BPSD (better stated as ecobiopsychosocial) can include a wide array of interventions including behavioral, environmental, and caregiver supportive interventions.[30] Ecobiopsychosocial treatments are endorsed by multiple professional societies as first-line treatment for management of BPSD including the American Psychiatric Association, American Geriatrics Society, and American Association for Geriatric Psychiatry.[31,32] However, this has not been translated to real-world care because of many factors including lack of provider training, time required to implement interventions, lack of reimbursement, and heterogeneity of interventions.[7] Behavioral interventions targeted at the person with dementia may include reminiscence therapy (discussion of past experiences), aromatherapy, Snoezelen (soothing and stimulating environment), and acupuncture.[33,34] Studies have demonstrated inconsistent support for the overall efficacy of these interventions in reducing BPSD.[35] Behavioral interventions focused on the environment may include correcting overstimulation or understimulation, addressing safety problems, increasing activity and structure, and establishing routine. There has been growing evidence for the role of the environment in preventing and reducing behaviors but there are few randomized controlled trials.[36]

The behavioral interventions with the most evidence to support reduction in BPSD are caregiver-supportive interventions. These interventions typically include problem-solving with the caregiver to identify modifiable causes of behaviors and enhanced communication between the patient and caregiver dyad. A meta-analysis of 23 randomized controlled trials with family caregiver interventions found these interventions significantly reduced BPSD, with an effect size greater than that for antipsychotics for agitation/aggression or cognitive enhancers for cognitive symptoms.[37]

THE DESCRIBE, INVESTIGATE, CREATE, EVALUATE APPROACH

The Describe, Investigate, Create, Evaluate (DICE) approach is an assessment and management algorithm created by a national multidisciplinary expert panel. Using an organized assessment approach or algorithm, such as DICE, can help providers integrate prevention, assessment, and management of BPSD.[38] The DICE approach can assist providers and caregivers in evaluation and management of BPSD and includes consideration of possible etiologies, includes caregivers, integrates pharmacologic and nonpharmacologic interventions, and has flexibility to use in various care settings (**Fig. 2**). To expand on and detail the DICE approach it is helpful to consider the following case example:

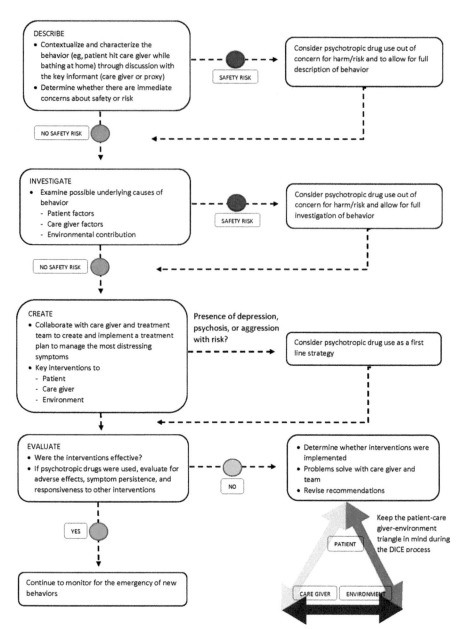

Fig. 2. The DICE approach. (*Adapted from* Kales HC, Gitlin LN, Lyketsos CG. Assessment and management of behavioral and psychological symptoms of dementia. BMJ 2015;350:h369; with permission.)

Mr N is a 65-year-old married man with a history of early onset Alzheimer disease. He lives at home with his wife who is 55 years old and serves as his primary caregiver. He began experiencing memory loss 5 years ago and a recent Montreal Cognitive Assessment was 10 out of 30. His wife reports lately Mr N has been irritable and verbally aggressive. His wife feels as though she is "walking on eggshells." His primary care physician refers Mr N to see a geriatric psychiatrist, requesting a medication to calm Mr N down.

Step 1: Describe

The first step of the DICE approach is to gather a detailed description of the problematic behavior and the context in which it occurs. This may involve a discussion with the patient's caregiver and patient with dementia if possible to understand the behaviors of concerns, identify antecedents, and other potentially modifiable factors. A full description of behavior goes beyond "agitation" (which, it can be argued is as nonspecific as "shortness of breath") and gives a full contextual picture (who, what, why, when, where). Thus, with such a full description, "agitation" becomes "anxiety and resistance to getting a daily bath" and leads directly to possible underlying causes in Step 2.

In the case of Mr N we would want to talk with his wife to better understand the behaviors that are most concerning. His wife reports Mr N has been verbally aggressive yelling "Leave me alone!" on a daily basis. He has never been physically aggressive toward his wife but she feels intimidated at times. These episodes of verbal aggression often occur when trying to get Mr N to medical appointments or take a daily bath. When asked, Mr N is not aware of these episodes. His wife states that she is stressed trying to take care of Mr N and she has had to take over all household responsibilities.

Step 2: Investigate

In the investigate stage, it is important to evaluate the possible causes of the problem behaviors. Patient-related factors, such as medication side effects, pain, medical conditions, and boredom, may be driving such behaviors. Caregiver factors related to a mismatch between caregiver expectations and patient capabilities, poor communication, or caregiver burden may contribute to behaviors. Lastly, environmental causes, such as changes in home environment and overstimulation or understimulation, may be contributing.

On examination, we note that Mr N is very hard of hearing with his wife stating he often refuses to wear his hearing aids and hides them throughout the house. He continues to rub his shoulder throughout the examination, which his wife believes may be related to an old rotator cuff injury. His wife describes that he often refuses care tasks, such as bathing, stating, "I think he does this just to make me upset." His wife acknowledges feeling "completely burnt out," feeling guilty asking her family for more assistance. She admits when stressed her communication style can be negative and scolding. When asked about the daily routine, Mr N spends most of his day at home watching television while his wife babysits the grandchildren. Previously an avid golfer and runner, Mr N now has limited activity and exercise during the day.

Step 3: Create

In the create stage the provider, caregiver, and team collaborate to create and implement a treatment plan. This could include responding to physical problems, improving communication with patient/caregiver dyad, and ensuring that the environment is safe.

For Mr N, we rule out any acute medical issues that may be contributing to his symptoms, such as a urinary tract infection. Additionally, we coordinate with his primary care physician to allow for more optimal control of his shoulder pain; this may include a standing dose of a pain medication for a time because he may forget or not be able to ask for an as-needed medication dose. We should also try to ensure that he is wearing his hearing aids. Given Mr N's previous level of physical activity, we work toward structuring routine and activities during the day that are meaningful to him and tailored to his interests. His wife is provided with education regarding BPSD and calm communication approaches. We teach her to "relax the rules," suggesting that bathing does not need to occur daily. We prescribe respite services and try to get Mr N's family more involved, encouraging his wife to take care of her own medical and mental health needs.

Step 4: Evaluate

Lastly, providers and caregivers work to evaluate whether the interventions developed in the "create stage" have been implemented by the caregiver and are safe and effective. Any unintended side effects or consequences of the interventions should be brought to the patients' provider and new techniques can be trialed.

In the evaluation stage, we assess changes to Mr N's behaviors once his pain is better controlled and routine is structured into the day. We discuss with his wife which interventions were most helpful, which interventions failed to improve symptoms, and whether any unintended consequences or side effects were noted with any of the biopsychosocial interventions.

PLACE OF PSYCHOTROPICS IN DESCRIBE, INVESTIGATE, CREATE, EVALUATE APPROACH

Currently there are no FDA-approved pharmacotherapies for treatment of BPSD. However, psychotropic medications are often prescribed off-label for primary treatment of BPSD.[39] Current psychotropic medication classes most commonly used in BPSD include antipsychotics, antidepressants, anticonvulsants (including valproic acid and derivatives), benzodiazepines, and cholinesterase inhibitors. Although in real-world settings such medications are often used first line and choice is targeted to the symptom cluster that is most problematic (eg, use of antidepressants for treatment of depression, antipsychotics for treatment of delusions or agitation, and anticonvulsants for mood lability), such practice is decidedly not evidence based (eg, there is no evidence for the symptom cluster approach or for the efficacy of such medications as valproic acid and derivatives for BPSD). Psychotropic medications should be considered first line if imminent risk is present for (1) major depression with or without suicidal ideation, (2) psychosis causing harm or potential for harm, and (3) aggression with risk to self or others.[38] Psychotropic medications rarely help for such behaviors as unfriendliness, poor self-care, memory problems, inattention/apathy, repetitive verbalizations, and wandering.[7]

Antipsychotics

Of the agents used to treat BPSD, antipsychotics do have the strongest evidence base, although the effect size is moderate (0.13–0.16).[7] The largest trial evaluating antipsychotic use in patients with dementia, the Clinical Antipsychotic Trial of Intervention Effectiveness-Alzheimer's Disease (CATIE-AD) trial, of 421 subjects with psychosis, aggression, or agitation failed to find improved outcomes over placebo.[40] The 2005 and 2008 black box warnings were based on findings of a 1.6- to 1.7-fold increase in mortality for antipsychotics as compared with placebo in patients with dementia.[26,29] Antipsychotic medications are associated with other side effects including cognitive worsening, somnolence, abnormal gait/falls, and stroke.[41] QTc prolongation, metabolic effects (weight gain, dyslipidemia, diabetes), and movement disorders (parkinsonism, dystonia, tardive dyskinesia) are additional concerns.[42]

Prescribing of antipsychotic medications for BPSD follows the general prescribing principles for geriatric psychiatry: "start low and go slow." Starting doses of antipsychotic medications are generally one-fourth to one-half of typical starting doses for adults (**Table 2**). For patients with Parkinson disease dementia or Lewy body dementia, special caution is required with use of antipsychotic medications because these patients are sensitive to the motor side effects of antipsychotic medications.[7] In these patients preference is given to use of cholinesterase inhibitors, such as rivastigmine, as first-line treatment of BPSD.[43] For patients who fail to respond to cholinesterase inhibitors, preferred agents included quetiapine and clozapine given lower blockade of the dopamine 2 receptor and less risk for extrapyramidal side effects, although these medications are still associated with increased mortality.[44] In 2016 pimavanserin was approved by the FDA for treatment of Parkinson disease psychosis.[45] This antipsychotic has a novel mechanism of action with no appreciable dopamine 2 blockade or risk for extrapyramidal symptoms, working as a selective inverse agonist at the serotonin 2A receptor.[46] However, pimavanserin still carries the same black box warning for increased mortality in use with patients with dementia and can cause QT prolongation.

Antidepressants

Antidepressant medications may have efficacy for treating agitation but have not shown consistent benefits for treating depression in dementia over five randomized controlled trials.[47] Antidepressant mediations are also associated with adverse events including sleep changes, nausea, vomiting, hyponatremia, and potential for QT prolongation with citalopram.[7] Low doses of the antidepressant trazodone (12.5–25 mg) can be used at times for treatment of agitation and anxiety in lieu of antipsychotic medication or benzodiazepines. In 2014 the Citalopram for Agitation in Alzheimer Disease (CITAD) study randomized patients to receive citalopram, finding patients treated with citalopram had significant improvements in agitation, caregiver stress, improved performance of activities of daily living, and reduction in use of a rescue medication (lorazepam) as compared with placebo.[48] However, patients treated with citalopram were found to also have worsening cognition and QT prolongation, which may limit its use.

Anticonvulsants

Available studies evaluating use of anticonvulsants, such as valproic acid, have not shown clear evidence for benefit and are associated with increased risk of mortality.[49,50] Two small studies looking at carbamazepine showed some benefit for treatment of agitation.[51,52] However, these medications are associated with serious risks including hepatitis, pancreatitis, and thrombocytopenia for valproic acid, and agranulocytosis and pancytopenia for carbamazepine.[53] Anticonvulsant agents are helpful at

Table 2
Starting and dose range of atypical antipsychotics for treatment of behavioral and psychological symptoms of dementia

Antipsychotic	Starting Dose	Dose Range
Risperidone	0.25–0.5 mg q h	0.25–2 mg/d
Quetiapine	12.5–25 q h	25–600 mg/d
Olanzapine	1.25–5 mg q h	2.5–20 mg/d
Aripiprazole	1–2 mg daily	2.5–20 mg/d
For Lewy body dementia or Parkinson disease dementia		
Quetiapine or clozapine	6.25–12.5 mg	25–350 mg/d

times at addressing mood instability and in the setting of prolonged QT where antipsychotic medications should be avoided.

Benzodiazepines

The use of benzodiazepines is associated with significant risks including increased cognitive impairment, disinhibition, falls, sedation, and respiratory suppression.[54] Given the lack of evidence of supporting use of benzodiazepines over placebo or other medications, use is not recommend outside of an acute behavioral crisis.[55,56]

Cholinesterase Inhibitors and Memantine

Cholinesterase inhibitors and memantine are the primary treatment of the cognitive symptoms of Alzheimer disease. However, some studies have suggested that these medications may also help to alleviated BPSD. A systematic review of cholinesterase inhibitors found a significant although small reduction in BPSD (overall reduction of 1.72 points on the 120-point neuropsychiatric inventory).[57] Studies for use of memantine have been equally mixed, with a recent trial demonstrating no benefit over placebo in reducing agitation in Alzheimer disease.[58] Cholinesterase inhibitors are associated with gastrointestinal side effects, such as diarrhea, nausea, and vomiting, and symptomatic bradycardia.[59] Side effects of memantine include headache, confusion, and dizziness.[60]

SUMMARY

Although cognitive impairment is the hallmark of dementia, behavioral disturbances are universally experienced by people with dementia throughout the course of the illness. BPSD causes a significant negative impact on quality of life, health care outcomes, caregiver stress/burden, and health care costs. However, treatment of BPSD may help to change the trajectory for patients and their caregivers. Nonpharmacologic treatments have been recommended as first-line treatment of BPSD by multiple professional organizations and expert panels and should target patient with dementia factors, caregiver factors, and environmental factors. Despite no medications having an FDA indication for management of BPSD, psychotropic medications are often prescribed off-label without significant evidence to support their use. The DICE approach can provide a structured method to investigate and treat BPSD with flexibility to use in multiple treatment settings. Treating clinicians need to consider the full biopsychosocial complexity of BPSD to best approach and guide care.

REFERENCES

1. Alzheimer's Association. 2016 Alzheimer's disease facts and figures. Alzheimers Dement 2016;12:459–509.
2. Hebert LE, Weuve J, Scherr PA, et al. Alzheimer disease in the United States (2010-2050) estimated using the 2010 census. Neurology 2013;80:1778–83.
3. Schulz R, Patterson TL. Caregiving in geriatric psychiatry. Am J Geriatr Psychiatry 2004;12:234–7.
4. Friedman EM, Shih RA, Langa KM, et al. US prevalence and predictors of informal caregiving for dementia. Health Aff (Millwood) 2015;34:1637–41.
5. Lyketsos CG, Carrillo MC, Ryan JM, et al. Neuropsychiatric symptoms in Alzheimer's disease. Alzheimers Dement 2011;7:532–9.
6. Steinberg M, Hess K, Corcoran C, et al. Vascular risk factors and neuropsychiatric symptoms in Alzheimer's disease: the Cache County Study. Int J Geriatr Psychiatry 2014;29:153–9.

7. Kales HC, Gitlin LN, Lyketsos CG. Assessment and management of behavioral and psychological symptoms of dementia. BMJ 2015;350:h369.
8. Rose KC, Gitlin LN. Background characteristics and treatment-related factors associated with treatment success or failure in a non-pharmacological intervention for dementia caregivers. Int Psychogeriatr 2017;29:1005–14.
9. Lyketsos CG, Lopez O, Jones B, et al. Prevalence of neuropsychiatric symptoms in dementia and mild cognitive impairment: results from the cardiovascular health study. JAMA 2002;288:1475–83.
10. Rabins PV, Schwartz S, Black BS, et al. Predictors of progression to severe Alzheimer's disease in an incidence sample. Alzheimers Dement 2013;9:204–7.
11. Wancata J, Windhaber J, Krautgartner M, et al. The consequences of non-cognitive symptoms of dementia in medical hospital departments. Int J Psychiatry Med 2003;33:257–71.
12. Yaffe K, Fox P, Newcomer R, et al. Patient and caregiver characteristics and nursing home placement in patients with dementia. JAMA 2002;287:2090–7.
13. Clyburn LD, Stones MJ, Hadjistavropoulos T, et al. Predicting caregiver burden and depression in Alzheimer's disease. J Gerontol B Psychol Sci Soc Sci 2000; 55:S2–13.
14. Beeri MS, Werner P, Davidson M, et al. The cost of behavioral and psychological symptoms of dementia (BPSD) in community dwelling Alzheimer's disease patients. Int J Geriatr Psychiatry 2002;17:403–8.
15. Geda YE, Schneider LS, Gitlin LN, et al. Neuropsychiatric symptoms in Alzheimer's disease: past progress and anticipation of the future. Alzheimers Dement 2013;9:602–8.
16. Hodgson NA, Gitlin LN, Winter L, et al. Undiagnosed illness and neuropsychiatric behaviors in community residing older adults with dementia. Alzheimer Dis Assoc Disord 2011;25:109–15.
17. Gerlach LB, Kales HC. Learning their language: the importance of detecting and managing pain in dementia. Am J Geriatr Psychiatry 2017;25:155–7.
18. Husebo BS, Ballard C, Sandvik R, et al. Efficacy of treating pain to reduce behavioural disturbances in residents of nursing homes with dementia: cluster randomised clinical trial. BMJ 2011;343:d4065.
19. von Gunten A, Pcnet C, Rossier J. The impact of personality characteristics on the clinical expression in neurodegenerative disorders: a review. Brain Res Bull 2009;80:179–91.
20. Norton MJ, Allen RS, Snow AL, et al. Predictors of need-driven behaviors in nursing home residents with dementia and associated certified nursing assistant burden. Aging Ment Health 2010;14:303–9.
21. Pinquart M, Sörensen S. Differences between caregivers and noncaregivers in psychological health and physical health: a meta-analysis. Psychol Aging 2003;18:250–67.
22. de Vugt ME, Nicolson NA, Aalten P, et al. Behavioral problems in dementia patients and salivary cortisol patterns in caregivers. J Neuropsychiatry Clin Neurosci 2005;17:201–7.
23. Smith M, Hall GR, Gerdner L, et al. Application of the progressively lowered stress threshold model across the continuum of care. Nurs Clin North Am 2006;41:57–81.
24. Schneider LS, Pollock VE, Lyness SA. A metaanalysis of controlled trials of neuroleptic treatment in dementia. J Am Geriatr Soc 1990;38:553–63.

25. Yury CA, Fisher JE. Meta-analysis of the effectiveness of atypical antipsychotics for the treatment of behavioural problems in persons with dementia. Psychother Psychosom 2007;76:213–8.

26. US Food and Drug Administration. Deaths with antipsychotics in elderly patients with behavioral disturbances. 2005. Available at: https://www.fda.gov/drugs/drugsafety/postmarketdrugsafetyinformationforpatientsandproviders/ucm053171. Accessed May 5, 2017.

27. Gill SS, Bronskill SE, Normand SL, et al. Antipsychotic drug use and mortality in older adults with dementia. Ann Intern Med 2007;146:775–86.

28. Schneeweiss S, Setoguchi S, Brookhart A, et al. Risk of death associated with the use of conventional versus atypical antipsychotic drugs among elderly patients. CMAJ 2007;176:627–32.

29. US Food and Drug Administration. Information for Healthcare Professionals: Conventional Antipsychotics. 2008. Available at: https://www.fda.gov/Drugs/DrugSafety/PostmarketDrugSafetyInformationforPatientsandProviders/ucm124830.htm. Accessed May 5, 2017.

30. Cohen-Mansfield J. Nonpharmacologic interventions for psychotic symptoms in dementia. J Geriatr Psychiatry Neurol 2003;16:219–24.

31. American Geriatrics Society, American Association of Geriatric Psychiatry. Consensus statement on improving the quality of mental health care in U.S. nursing homes: management of depression and behavioral symptoms associated with dementia. J Am Geriatr Soc 2003;51:1287–98.

32. Choosing wisely. Five things physicians and patients should question. Arlington (VA): American Psychiatric Association; 2013. Available at: http://www.choosingwisely.org/societies/american-psychiatric-association/. Accessed May 21, 2017.

33. Burns A, Perry E, Holmes C, et al. A double-blind placebo-controlled randomized trial of Melissa officinalis oil and donepezil for the treatment of agitation in Alzheimer's disease. Dement Geriatr Cogn Disord 2011;31:158–64.

34. Chung JC, Lai CK, Chung PM, et al. Snoezelen for dementia. Cochrane Database Syst Rev 2002;(4):CD003152.

35. O'Neil M, Freeman M, Christensen V. Non-pharmacological interventions for behavioral symptoms of dementia: a systematic review of the evidence. VA-ESP Project #05-225; 2011.

36. Gitlin LN, Liebman J, Winter L. Are environmental interventions effective in the management of Alzheimer's disease and related disorders?: a synthesis of the evidence. Alzheimers Care Today 2003;4:85–107.

37. Brodaty H, Arasaratnam C. Meta-analysis of nonpharmacological interventions for neuropsychiatric symptoms of dementia. Am J Psychiatry 2012;169:946–53.

38. Kales HC, Gitlin LN, Lyketsos CG. Management of neuropsychiatric symptoms of dementia in clinical settings: recommendations from a multidisciplinary expert panel. J Am Geriatr Soc 2014;62:762–9.

39. Jeste DV, Blazer D, Casey D, et al. ACNP white paper: update on use of antipsychotic drugs in elderly persons with dementia. Neuropsychopharmacology 2008; 33:957–70.

40. Schneider LS, Tariot PN, Dagerman KS, et al. Effectiveness of atypical antipsychotic drugs in patients with Alzheimer's disease. N Engl J Med 2006;355: 1525–38.

41. Douglas IJ, Smeeth L. Exposure to antipsychotics and risk of stroke: self controlled case series study. BMJ 2008;337:a1227.

42. American Diabetes Association, American Psychiatric Association, American Association of Clinical Endocrinologists, et al. Consensus development conference

on antipsychotic drugs and obesity and diabetes. J Clin Psychiatry 2004;65: 267–72.

43. Rolinski M, Fox C, Maidment I, et al. Cholinesterase inhibitors for dementia with Lewy bodies, Parkinson's disease dementia and cognitive impairment in Parkinson's disease. Cochrane Database Syst Rev 2012;3:CD006504.

44. Weintraub D, Chiang C, Kim HM, et al. Association of antipsychotic use with mortality risk in patients with Parkinson Disease. JAMA Neurol 2016;73:535–41.

45. Mathis MV, Muoio BM, Andreason P, et al. The US Food and Drug Administration's perspective on the new antipsychotic pimavanserin. J Clin Psychiatry 2017;78: e668–73.

46. Cruz MP. Pimavanserin (Nuplazid): a treatment for hallucinations and delusions associated with Parkinson's disease. P T 2017;42:368–71.

47. Seitz DP, Adunuri N, Gill SS, et al. Antidepressants for agitation and psychosis in dementia. Cochrane Database Syst Rev 2011;(2):CD008191.

48. Porsteinsson AP, Drye LT, Pollock BG, et al. Effect of citalopram on agitation in Alzheimer disease: the CitAD randomized clinical trial. JAMA 2014;311:682–91.

49. Konovalov S, Muralee S, Tampi RR. Anticonvulsants for the treatment of behavioral and psychological symptoms of dementia: a literature review. Int Psychogeriatr 2008;20:293–308.

50. Maust DT, Kim HM, Seyfried LS, et al. Antipsychotics, other psychotropics, and the risk of death in patients with dementia: number needed to harm. JAMA Psychiatry 2015;72:438–45.

51. Tariot PM, Erb R, Podgorski CA, et al. Efficacy and tolerability of carbamazepine for agitation and aggression in dementia. Am J Psychiatry 1998;155:54–61.

52. Olin JT, Fox LS, Pawluczyk S, et al. A pilot randomized trial of carbamazepine for behavioral symptoms in treatment-resistant outpatients with Alzheimer disease. Am J Geriatr Psychiatry 2001;9:400–5.

53. Dols A, Sienaert P, van Gerven H, et al. The prevalence and management of side effects of lithium and anticonvulsants as mood stabilizers in bipolar disorder from a clinical perspective: a review. Int Clin Psychopharmacol 2013;28:287–96.

54. Peisah C, Chan DK, McKay R, et al. Practical guidelines for the acute emergency sedation of the severely agitated older patient. Intern Med J 2011;41:651–7.

55. Christensen DB, Benfield WR. Alprazolam as an alternative to low-dose haloperidol in older, cognitively impaired nursing facility patients. J Am Geriatr Soc 1998; 46:620–5.

56. Meehan KM, Wang H, David SR, et al. Comparison of rapidly acting intramuscular olanzapine, lorazepam, and placebo: a double-blind, randomized study in acutely agitated patients with dementia. Neuropsychopharmacology 2002; 26:494–504.

57. Trinh NH, Hoblyn J, Mohanty S, et al. Efficacy of cholinesterase inhibitors in the treatment of neuropsychiatric symptoms and functional impairment in Alzheimer disease: a meta-analysis. JAMA 2003;289:210–6.

58. Fox C, Crugel M, Maidment I, et al. Efficacy of memantine for agitation in Alzheimer's dementia: a randomised double-blind placebo controlled trial. PLoS One 2012;7:e35185.

59. Kaduszkiewicz H, Zimmermann T, Beck-Bornholdt HP, et al. Cholinesterase inhibitors for patients with Alzheimer's disease: systematic review of randomised clinical trials. BMJ 2005;331:321–7.

60. McShane R, Areosa Sastre A, Minakaran N. Memantine for dementia. Cochrane Database Syst Rev 2006;(2):CD003154.

Palliative Care for Dementia

Jonathan T. Stewart, MD[a,b,*], Susan K. Schultz, MD[a]

KEYWORDS

• End of life • Palliative care • Hospice • Dementia • Dying

KEY POINTS

• The population with dementia will represent a group with specific end-of-life care needs that will require better access to hospice and palliative services.
• End-of-life care in dementia has special considerations in addressing behavioral disturbances and maintaining attention to goals of care.
• Unique problems in the care of the patient with dementia at the end of life may be related to refractory delirium (confusion) and cachexia (failure to maintain weight).

INTRODUCTION

With the increase of the elderly population and increasing burden of dementia care, one may consider the need for palliative and hospice services as an urgent public health priority, particularly given that Alzheimer's disease is now the sixth leading cause of death in the United States.[1] This public health need is underscored by the severe burden of emotional distress endured by family caregivers and the potential for relief afforded by appropriate end-of-life services in dementia.[2,3] End-of-life services have been historically created for the context of cancer care, with less of a focus on dementia, although this has changed considerably in recent years. For example, in 1995, less than 1% of hospice patients were observed to have a primary diagnosis of dementia,[4] whereas almost 15% of all hospice enrollments in 2014 were in the context of dementia care.[5] Despite this reassuring rapid increase, there remain challenges in ensuring that patients with dementia are given the chance for the best possible care at the end of life.

Disclosure: The authors have nothing to disclose.
[a] Psychiatry, James A. Haley Veterans Hospital, University of South Florida College of Medicine, 13000 Bruce B Downs Boulevard, Tampa, FL 33612, USA; [b] Geriatric Medicine, James A. Haley Veterans Hospital, University of South Florida College of Medicine, 13000 Bruce B Downs Boulevard, Tampa, FL 33612, USA
* Corresponding author. Psychiatry Service, James A Haley VA Hospital, 116A, 13000 Bruce B Downs Boulevard, Tampa, FL 33612.
E-mail address: jonathan.stewart1@va.gov

Psychiatr Clin N Am 41 (2018) 141–151
https://doi.org/10.1016/j.psc.2017.10.011
0193-953X/18/Published by Elsevier Inc.

psych.theclinics.com

Management of dementia is complicated by neuropsychiatric symptoms such that the longitudinal care of a psychiatrist or other mental health provider is often a central part of the primary care of the patient and a major source of family support. Given the importance of continuity of care at the end of life, the involvement of psychiatry in palliative and hospice services affords a critical opportunity for growth. For example, a recent European consensus document has outlined recommendations for optimal palliative care for dementia and included continuity of services as among its top major domains of high-quality care.[6] Further, within the top domain, an explicit recommendation included attention to behavioral care within a comprehensive care setting. To achieve the best care for both our patients suffering from dementia as well as their caregivers, it is necessary to achieve 2 goals, one is to improve access for persons with dementia, and the second is to engage providers with psychiatry expertise to be involved in those services. This article addresses how issues in prognostication in dementia may affect the first goal. The article then reviews how psychiatry expertise may be used for the specific clinical issues that require attention in dementia care at the end of life.

PROGNOSTICATION

Difficulties with prognostication is one of the greatest barriers to access to end-of-life services in the content of dementia, given the absence of highly predictable metrics in estimating survival relative to other medical conditions.[7–10] The lack of clear metrics and variable outcomes in survival time creates significant difficulty for families, patients, and even clinical care providers to conceptualize dementia as a terminal condition.[11,12] The recent European consensus notes in its primary recommendation that dementia can realistically be regarded as a terminal condition and "recognizing its eventual terminal nature is the basis for anticipating future problems and an impetus to the provision of adequate palliative care."[6] Although there is great heterogeneity in its early stages, all dementias move toward a stereotypic terminal stage of inexorable functional decline, frailty, cachexia, and medical complications, with median survival about 5 years from diagnosis.[11] In this regard, end-stage dementia is strikingly similar to advanced cancer or congestive heart failure. One means of conceptualizing end-stage dementia is a condition of "brain failure," with all the characteristics associated with other major organ failure (eg, advanced liver failure or congestive heart failure).[13] When viewed as progressive major organ failure, it may help to reduce the likelihood of inappropriately viewing dementia as purely a deficit in memory function, which does not adequately reflect the global dysfunction and deterioration of advanced disease.

Traditionally, the course of end-stage dementia has been characterized as one of slow, steady decline, but Sachs and colleagues[7] have suggested that the more likely scenario is one of slow progression punctuated by recurrent health crises. In this regard, the actual pattern may be more akin to that seen in end-stage chronic obstructive pulmonary disease or congestive heart failure, where small disruptions in health status may result in severe symptoms. The crises seen in end-stage dementia may be more variable given that there is a risk for instability in the face of minor perturbations in fluid status, infections, or aspiration. Consequently, these crises may include episodes of aspiration pneumonia, urosepsis, dehydration, delirium, or falls. Medical decision making gains importance during these crises and the importance of a palliative approach comes to the fore when there is a risk for aggressive interventions (hospitalization, artificial nutrition and hydration). Recurrent crises offer an important opportunity to engage with the patient and family decision makers about appropriate expectations and prognosis. The importance of the appropriate goals of care is a pressing issue that requires diligence among care providers to avoid recurrent hospitalizations and their potential adverse consequences. It has been shown within the last decade that there has been a progressive increase in the number of nursing home patients dying in the hospital as opposed to remaining in place,[14] reflecting a potential breakdown in communication and lack of attention to patient-centered care given that acute hospitalization is likely to be incongruent with goals of care that take into account prognosis in advanced dementia.

Prognostic criteria for survival in dementia have been documented by the National Hospice and Palliative Care Organization.[15] According to these criteria, a patient is likely to die within 6 months if at Functional Assessment Staging stage 7 and with 1 or more listed medical or nutritional complications. Functional Assessment Staging stage 7 is characterized by dependence in all activities of daily living, incontinence of bowel and bladder, and speech limited to no more than 6 usable words. Medical complications may include aspiration pneumonia, upper urinary tract infection, recurrent sepsis, or stage III or IV pressure ulcers; nutritional complications include greater than 10% weight loss in the past 6 months or a serum albumin of less than 2.5 g/dL. These concepts have been adapted for use in determining eligibility for Medicare benefits. It has been observed that Medicare expenditures for dementia, particularly for patients in nursing homes, have increased dramatically over the last several years, and a recent analysis noted that nearly one-half of the recipients in nursing home care receiving hospice services were diagnosed with dementia, whereas another 10% had both dementia and cancer, suggesting that dementia is now comprising a large portion of hospice care recipients, particularly among nursing home patients.[16]

Although not used in Medicare benefit determination, Mitchell and colleagues[16] have developed the Mortality Risk Index, which has been shown to have greater predictive value than the National Hospice and Palliative Care Organization criteria in a large nursing home cohort, although it has not been validated in non–nursing home populations. The Mortality Risk Index is a weighted composite of 12 items taken from the Minimum Data Set, a standard database collected on all nursing home residents in US nursing homes that receive federal funds. As the public health significance of end-stage dementia care grows to consume more health care expenditures, prognostic work along these lines will likely assume greater importance. For example, there are other robust predictors of 6-month mortality reported in advanced dementia; one especially ominous predictor is the presence of a new hip fracture.[17,18]

PLANNING

Although caregiver education remains a cornerstone of managing dementia, education about prognosis and goals of care remains an opportunity for growth. For example, Mitchell and colleagues[19] reported that only 18% of families of individuals with dementia had ever discussed prognosis with a physician. This is concerning, given that Mitchell and associates[19] also reported that education about prognosis was associated with a lower incidence of aggressive interventions at the end of life, such as tube feeding and hospitalization. Patient and family education regarding advanced directives should start early and should be continually tailored to anticipated problems on the horizon. Fortunately, recent work has attended to developing structured tools to aid clinicians in having the necessary conversations to develop a patient-centered treatment plan that is appropriate for expectations and prognosis. The Goals of Care intervention[20] has recently been evaluated in a population of end-stage dementia with an average age of 86.5 years. The intervention included a video decision aid program and structured meeting to discuss the treatment and care plan for the decision makers of the individuals with dementia. It was shown that the Goals of Care decision aid intervention improved end-of-life communication and reduced by nearly one-half the number of hospital transfers when compared with other patients and increased the likelihood of palliative care recommendations in the care plan. Although this is just one example of a targeted effort to optimize end-of-life care, the role of the psychiatrist is perhaps ideally suited to help disseminate and enhance this type of structured communication practice.

Standardized advance directive documents offer an existing format to begin a conversation regarding goals of care; however, they are often not adequate for patients with dementia because they may not address common scenarios such as placement of a feeding tube or foregoing of antibiotics or hospitalization,[13] and it is best to incorporate these preferences into the document after a thorough discussion of likely risks and limited benefits of such interventions. The discussion may be quite difficult emotionally for the patient and especially the family; therefore, it is essential to compassionately explore the underlying feelings and beliefs behind these preferences as well as emphasize that goals of care should focus on what the patient would choose as opposed to the surrogates' preferences (ie, substituted judgment).

DELIRIUM

Dementia is the most consistently reported risk factor for incident delirium and likely the most pressing behavioral disturbance as the dementia progresses.[21] Delirium can be a challenge to identify in end-stage dementia owing to numerous overlapping features. The Confusion Assessment Method described by Inouye and colleagues[22] identifies 4 key features of delirium: decreased attention, acute onset and fluctuating course, disorganized thought, and altered level of consciousness. Patients with end-stage dementia often seem to be inattentive and difficult to engage, and formal testing of attention is generally impossible. Likewise, it will be impossible to identify disorganization of thought in a patient with little or no language, and lethargy and hypersomnia are very common in the last few months of life. This leaves only 1 feature, acute onset and perhaps fluctuating course, to suggest the presence of a superimposed delirium. In the advanced dementia population, delirium can present with a wide variety of acute behavioral changes or decreases in already limited function. Even the abrupt change in mental status may fail to provide diagnostic value in the context of frailty and dementia, as it is increasingly recognized that particularly after acute care interventions, elderly adults may suffer a protracted delirium that persists over several months, supporting the importance of avoiding acute hospitalizations among advanced patients with dementia. For example, Kiely and colleagues[23] demonstrated in a large sample of delirious elderly patients seen acutely in hospital settings that, on longitudinal evaluation, one-third were still exhibiting delirium 6 months later and that persistent delirium was a significant predictor of mortality. When examining premorbid predictors, it was shown that 38% of the sample had a preexisting diagnosis of dementia before the acute care event.

This work illustrates the complex and deleterious effects of persistent confusion that may arise from multiple concurrent sources. Consequently, the differential diagnosis of delirium in the end-stage patient with dementia is quite broad and may include factors that are not remediable. Common etiologies include adverse drug effects, infection (eg, aspiration pneumonia), dehydration, hyponatremia, and a wide variety of acute or chronic medical conditions. A recent analysis of a national database of cases of delirium occurring among hospitalized persons with dementia between 1998 and 2005 observed that the overall prevalence of dementia-associated delirium actually decreased over time when considering all associated causes, but unfortunately the prevalence of drug-induced delirium was shown to increase over this time interval.[24] Although the cornerstone of delirium treatment is identification of the underlying etiology, in a hospice environment this will be highly dependent on the patient's ability to tolerate any evaluation, the likelihood of improving quality of life with treatment, and the life expectancy and goals of care that sometimes necessitate comfort medications.[13]

Regardless of whether the etiology may be fully evaluated or treated, the impact of the delirium on the patient's wellbeing requires attention. Hypoactive delirium is more common than agitated, hyperactive delirium in the last months of life[25] and there may be relatively lower distress and suffering in this scenario relative to agitated delirium. Although there are few studies in terminal illness, haloperidol remains the standard of practice when distressing symptoms require pharmacologic treatment.[26,27] The persistence of haloperidol as the practice standard is likely attributable to its low likelihood of autonomic adverse effects and can be given orally, subcutaneously, or intravenously. Extrapyramidal side effects infrequently limit treatment with antipsychotic medication, and can generally be addressed by lowering the dose or switching to an atypical agent. At present, there is a lack of comparative trials of atypical antipsychotics with haloperidol in the management of delirium, limiting conclusions regarding their relative efficacy. In general, consensus opinion suggests that haloperidol 1 to 2 mg orally every 2 to 4 hours may be appropriate for as needed management of delirium in the absence of frailty, with lower doses (0.25–0.5 mg) in the elderly or frail patient.[28] Other important measures include avoidance or camouflaging of distressing medical devices (eg, intravenous lines, indwelling urinary catheters, bed alarms), maintaining a relatively quiet and understimulating environment, maintaining a normal diurnal cycle of light intensity, and attending to fall risk and other safety issues.[26]

BEHAVIORAL PROBLEMS

At least 80% to 90% of patients with dementia develop behavioral and psychological problems at some point, and these problems are generally more prominent in more severe dementia.[29] Furthermore, there is evidence that behavioral problems change qualitatively as well as quantitatively as dementia progresses; for example, delusions and hallucinations may presently less frequently in severe and end-stage dementia, whereas resistiveness to care may become more common until the last few months of life.[26] Given that end-stage patients with dementia are often nonverbal and unable to communicate the source of distress, and almost any behavioral change or problem (eg, yelling, combativeness, crying) may be indicative of almost any type of distress (eg, pain, dyspnea, fearfulness, etc). Family members and nursing staff may recognize subtle cues and provide assistance as the first line behavioral observers.[13] In view of the close relationship between caregiver distress and behavioral symptoms in dementia, their concordance suggests that caregiver reporting of behaviors may be significantly influenced by their own distress, reflecting the importance of managing the dyad's needs together.[30] Resistiveness to care is a common behavioral problem in severe dementia, although in the context of disease progression at the end of life there is an emergence of lethargy and passivity.[26] In general, in the palliative care setting, in the absence of severe distress or agitation, the optimal approach is nonpharmacologic. Specific techniques that may be useful in the context of resistiveness to care include limiting the amount of hands-on care to that necessary to maintain comfort and quality of life, while avoiding needless stimulation. A minimalist approach to care with some pleasant distraction is ideal, with close attention to adherence to the patient's preferences and goals of care.

The cornerstone of managing behavioral problems is a concerted, interdisciplinary attempt to identify and remove sources of distress and identifying any unmet needs. It is often quite difficult to identify the problem with the limited information available. Challenges in optimizing treatment require a high level of communication with family members who know the patient well and can assist in maintaining patient-centered goals. For example, in a patient who has established wishes to avoid artificial hydration, there may be challenges in managing dehydration that require a commitment across the care team to focus on comfort and patient goals while at times permitting conditions such as low fluid intake to avoid unwanted aggressive care that increases distress. Maintaining patient-centered goals for comfort may also require intuitive clinical decision making in the absence of data from invasive tests or information from a cogent patient. Along these lines, given the difficulties in assessing pain in advanced dementia, some authors have advocated an empirical trial of analgesics (eg, routine acetaminophen or opioids) if no other source of distress can be identified.[31,32] Despite all efforts, it will sometimes be necessary to manage the patient's distress and agitation with antipsychotic medication if other efforts to reduce distress fail and the symptoms are persistent and harmful. There have been very few studies of pharmacotherapy for behavioral problems and distress in end-stage dementia, but the use of haloperidol as for delirium described is likely the most commonly used medication, although data regarding medication selection are severely limited.[9,26] One large study examined prescribing practices in nearly 300 patients, with a mean age of 86 years, admitted to hospice with progressive debility and weight loss.[33] Regarding antipsychotic medication, in this analysis the only agent observed to be commonly used was haloperidol, the most commonly prescribed drugs were acetaminophen, lorazepam, morphine, atropine, prochlorperazine, haloperidol, docusate, aspirin, and bisacodyl.[33]

PAIN AND DYSPNEA

Pain, either acute or chronic, is a common cause of suffering, agitation, and behavioral disturbance in patients with advanced dementia. Given the impaired ability of these patients to communicate needs, there is a high risk for pain to be undertreated or mistaken for a behavioral issue requiring antipsychotic treatment.[34,35] Even when detected, pain is often undertreated in patients with dementia, and this undertreatment has been shown to correlate with the severity of dementia.[36] Morrison and Siu[34] reported that in a cohort of patients with hip fracture, those with dementia received only one-third as much opioid analgesia as those without dementia, and that only 24% of those with dementia received any routine analgesics at all. This problem is of sufficient magnitude that several authors have recommended an empirical trial of analgesics for patients with behavioral problems for which no other etiology is found.[31,32] Recognition that pain is experienced in advanced dementia is essential to adequate treatment, with the recognition that the expression of pain is often atypical in dementia and complicated in advanced disease when patients nonverbal and unable to describe their experience.[37]

There are several rating scales for pain in nonverbal patients with dementia, including the Pain Assessment in Advanced Dementia Scale[38] and others,[35] which may be valuable tools to assist in pain assessment and follow-up within a comprehensive care setting. Pain, or presumptive pain, should always be addressed in this population and typically requires pharmacologic intervention. As a general rule, it is best to prescribe routinely scheduled, rather than as-needed, analgesics, because these patients will be unable to ask for as-needed medication.[37] Routine acetaminophen in doses up to 3000 mg/d may be effective for some patients where it can be tolerated with adverse effects. Opioids may cause some sedation initially in opioid-naive patients, but otherwise may be needed for adequate pain management with careful monitoring and adjustment for other medical conditions. One study demonstrated in a clinical sample that 75% of patients with dementia receiving palliative services were found to have clinically significant pain,[39] and of these 93% required treatment with morphine that resulted in pain control in the majority of the group with dementia. Dyspnea is also commonly seen in the late stages of all terminal illnesses, including dementia[40]; it may incur a significant burden of distress that may be alleviated through treatment with opioids.

ANOREXIA AND CACHEXIA

It is known that weight loss tends to occur with advancing age in all adults and intriguing research has shown that this problem may be accelerated substantially in the context of Alzheimer's dementia and may begin well before the onset of cognitive changes. In a longitudinal study of community older adults with and without cognitive changes, Kiely and colleagues[23] observed that the study participants weighted an average 6 to 8 pound less than their counterparts who did not proceed to a dementia diagnosis. Further, those who went on to have Alzheimer's disease experienced about 0.6 lbs of weight loss each year before diagnosis, which doubled to 1.2 lbs per year immediately before Alzheimer's detection. This observation of progressive weight decrease occurring before overt dementia is now a growing focus of attention, because it has been replicated in epidemiologic studies.[41] This observation suggests an underlying phenomenon that may be inherent to the illness that incurs a metabolic deficit. The relevance of this unusual metabolic change to potentially understanding fundamental pathogenic processes in dementia may yield important etiologic insights. Therefore, significant attention has been addressed toward the molecular underpinnings of this process, with the greatest potential likely incurred by dysregulation of leptin function.[42] Leptin plays a key role in multiple physiologic processes involved in neuronal function as well as adiposity and metabolic control, making it a likely mediator of weight in dementia throughout the course of the illness, including premorbidly. Additionally, after dementia has been diagnosed and the clinical illness has progressed, maintaining adequate oral intake and weight are well-known issues described in clinical practice.[43,44] There are a number of contributing factors, such as an inability to acquire or prepare food, anosmia, dysphagia, concurrent medical illness, adverse medication effects (eg, cholinesterase inhibitors), and inadequate diets.[13,45]

Like all end-stage diseases in the hospice setting, dementia is also associated with cachexia, a complex metabolic syndrome involving increased levels of proinflammatory cytokines that leads to chronic inflammation, muscle wasting, functional decline, and anorexia.[2] The development of cachexia in dementia represents an important problem that requires substantial education for family surrogate decision makers as well as allied staff to understand its complexity and lack of responsiveness to increased oral intake. The development of cachexia is a common final endpoint of advanced disease at the end of life[46] that is largely mediated by an increased catabolic and inflammatory state that has deleterious effects on muscle mass (inducing sarcopenia), as well as central nervous system effects that incur a loss of appetite (anorexia). Persistent inflammation further has deleterious effects on adipose tissue and hepatic function such that a continual release of acute phase reactants and other proinflammatory compounds ensues.[46] Although it may seem to be a solution, tube feeding and artificial nutrition have not been shown to improve health in dementia. Artificial feeling, such as via a percutaneous endoscopic gastrostomy tube, does not improve life expectancy, functional capacity, or quality of life, nor does it prevent aspiration pneumonia in advanced dementia.[47] Over the last 2 decades there has been a growing awareness of the lack of usefulness of enteral nutrition in end-stage dementia that has fortunately translated into clinical practices. Mitchell and colleagues[48] (2016) analyzed more than 71,000 patients in nursing homes with advanced dementia and dependence for eating between 2000 and 2014. During this time period, there was a 50% decrease in the proportion of patients receiving artificial nutrition. This encouraging finding likely attests to better communication between clinicians and families with greater adherence to goals of care. However, it is important to recognize that food has strong symbolic meaning in all cultures, and a family's efforts at providing comfort feeding and the interaction that it entails can be highly meaningful to patient and family alike. A reasonable approach[13] includes a search for treatable causes of anorexia (offending medications, dental problems, failure to respect longstanding food preferences, distraction or fearfulness during feeding, etc), encouraging family to try favorite or home-cooked foods; maintaining a pleasant, social but nondistracting atmosphere; providing continuous snacks; experimenting with food textures and temperatures; sweetening foods; and providing nutrient-dense supplements. It is often quite reasonable to forego dietary modifications designed to reduce aspiration risk (thickened liquids, for example) in favor of greater patient comfort and pleasure. Finally, there is limited evidence that appetite stimulants such as dronabinol or megestrol may modestly improve intake and quality of life, although improvement in function or life expectancy is rare.[43,44,48,49]

SUMMARY AND FUTURE DIRECTIONS

Hospice and palliative care for dementia is a relatively new area of study. As such, there are more questions than answers about how to best care for these most vulnerable patients. Hospice enrollment for end-stage dementia has improved dramatically over the past 2 decades, yet individuals continue to be referred to care within the last weeks or days of life. Improved prognostic skills and positive predictive models will be of great help in identifying those patients who will benefit most from hospice enrollment to ensure prompt referral. Once referred, many challenges remain in tailoring hospice care expertise for the special issues that distinguish the patient with dementia at the end of life. For example, the complex clinical and pathophysiologic interface between severe dementia and delirium remains a particularly fruitful area for future studies, as does the frequency and nature of cachexia. Such research will help the field reach perhaps the ultimate goal of maximal quality, comfort, and adherence to patients' wishes. A century ago when cure of most diseases was rarely possible, physicians were more focused on what always has been and always will be possible: presence and relief of suffering. Although most clinicians are adept at listing "reversible causes of dementia," it is clear that this effort only rarely succeeds in averting a course of cognitive decline and that cure is rare. Hospice and palliative medicine is recognizing the powerful role that it has in caring for the dementia population. Equipped with current knowledge, forethought, and compassion, we can go far in ensuring that our patients with dementia die with peace and dignity, leaving a positive legacy for those whom they leave behind.

REFERENCES

1. Alzheimer's Association. 2016 Alzheimer's disease facts and figures. Alzheimers Dement 2016;12:459–509.
2. Aminoff BZ, Adunsky A. Their last 6 months: suffering and survival of end-stage dementia patients. Age Ageing 2006;35:579–601.
3. Irwin SA, Mausbach BT, Koo D, et al. Association between hospice care and psychological outcomes in Alzheimer's spousal caregivers. J Palliat Med 2013;11:1450–4.
4. Hanrahan P, Luchins DJ. Feasible criteria for enrolling end-stage dementia patients in home hospice care. Hosp J 1995;10:47–54.
5. National Hospice and Palliative Care Organization Statistics, Available at: https://www.nhpco.org/sites/default/files/public/Statistics_Research/2015_Facts_Figures.pdf. Accessed April 20, 2017.
6. van der Steen JT, Helton MR, Ribbe MW. Prognosis is important in decisionmaking in Dutch nursing home patients with dementia and pneumonia. Int J Geriatr Psychiatry 2009;24:933–6.
7. Sachs GA, Shega JW, Cox-Hayley D. Barriers to excellent end-of-life care for patients with dementia. J Gen Intern Med 2004;19:1057–63.
8. Mitchell SL, Miller SC, Teno JM, et al. Prediction of 6-month survival of nursing home residents with advanced dementia using ADEPT vs hospice eligibility guidelines. JAMA 2010;304:1929–35.
9. Shuster JL. Palliative care for advanced dementia. Clin Geriatr Med 2000;16:373–86.
10. Sampson EL. Palliative care for people with dementia. Br Med Bull 2010;96:159–74.
11. Wolf-Klein G, Pekmezaris R, Chin L, et al. Conceptualizing Alzheimer's disease as a terminal medical illness. Am J Hosp Palliat Med 2007;24:77–82.
12. Hirot F. Palliative care for dementia patients. Geriatr Psychol Neuropsychiatr Vieil 2016;14:447–53.
13. Sekerak RJ, Stewart JT. Caring for the patient with endstage dementia. Ann Long Term Care 2014;22:36–43.
14. Temkin-Greener H, Zheng NT, Xing J, et al. Site of death among nursing home residents in the United States: changing patterns, 2003-2007. J Am Med Dir Assoc 2013;14(10):741–8.
15. Hospice Eligibility Requirements. Available at: https://www.nhpco.org/hospice-eligibility-requirements. Accessed April 14, 2017.
16. Gozalo P, Plotzke M, Mor V, et al. Changes in Medicare costs with the growth of hospice care in nursing homes. N Engl J Med 2015;372(19):1823–31.
17. Mitchell SL, Kiely DK, Hamel MB, et al. Estimating prognosis for nursing home residents with advanced dementia. JAMA 2004;291:2734–40.
18. Tarazona-Santabalbina FJ, Belenguer-Varea Á, Rovira Daudi E, et al. Severity of cognitive impairment as a prognostic factor for mortality and functional recovery of geriatric patients with hip fracture. Geriatr Gerontol Int 2015;15:289–95.
19. Mitchell SL, Teno JM, Kiely DK, et al. The clinical course of advanced dementia. N Engl J Med 2009;361:1529–38.
20. Rosemond C, Hanson LC, Zimmerman S. Goals of care or goals of trust? how family members perceive goals for dying nursing home residents. J Palliat Med 2017;20:360–5.

21. Boettger S, Jenewein J, Breitbart W. Delirium in advanced age and dementia: a prolonged refractory course of delirium and lower functional status. Palliat Support Care 2015;13:1113–21.
22. Inouye SK, van Dyck CH, Alessi CA, et al. Clarifying confusion: the confusion assessment method. A new method for detection of delirium. Ann Intern Med 1990;113:941–8.
23. Kiely DK, Marcantonio ER, Inouye SK, et al. Accelerated weight loss may precede diagnosis in Alzheimer disease. Arch Neurol 2006;9:1312–7.
24. Lin RY, Heacock LC, Fogel JF. Drug-induced, dementia-associated and non-dementia, non-drug delirium hospitalizations in the United States, 1998-2005: an analysis of the national inpatient sample. Drugs Aging 2010;27:51–61.
25. Breitbart W, Alici Y. Agitation and delirium at the end of life: "We couldn't manage him". JAMA 2008;300:2898–910.
26. Bush SH, Kanji S, Pereira JL, et al. Treating an established episode of delirium in palliative care: expert opinion and review of the current evidence base with recommendations for future development. J Pain Symptom Manage 2014;48: 231–48.
27. Stewart JT. Behavioral and emotional complications of neurologic disorders. In: Noseworthy JH, editor. Neurological therapeutics: principles and practice. 2nd edition. Abingdon (United Kingdom): Informa Healthcare; 2006. p. 3207–22.
28. Practice guideline for the treatment of patients with delirium. American Psychiatric Association. Am J Psychiatry 1999;156:1–20.
29. Brodaty H, Draper B, Saab D, et al. Psychosis, depression and behavioural disturbances in Sydney nursing home residents: prevalence and predictors. Int J Geriatr Psychiatry 2001;16:504–12.
30. Feast A, Orrell M, Russell I, et al. The contribution of caregiver psychosocial factors to distress associated with behavioural and psychological symptoms in dementia. Int J Geriatr Psychiatry 2017;32:76–85.
31. Snow AL, O'Malley KJ, Cody M, et al. A conceptual model of pain assessment for noncommunicative persons with dementia. Gerontologist 2004;44:807–17.
32. Volicer L. Management of severe Alzheimer's disease and end-of-life issues. Clin Geriatr Med 2001;17:377–91.
33. Sera L, Holmes HM, McPherson ML. Prescribing practices in hospice patients with adult failure to thrive or debility. Prog Palliat Care 2014;22:69–74.
34. Morrison RS, Siu AL. Survival in end-stage dementia following acute illness. JAMA 2000;284:47–52.
35. Zwakhalen SMG, Hamers JPH, Abu-Saad HH, et al. Pain in elderly people with severe dementia: a systematic review of behavioural pain assessment tools. BMC Geriatr 2006;6:3.
36. Scherder E, Oosterman J, Swaab D, et al. Recent developments in pain in dementia. BMJ 2005;330:461–4.
37. Haasum Y, Fastbom J, Fratiglioni L, et al. Pain treatment in elderly persons with and without dementia: a population-based study of institutionalized and home-dwelling elderly. Drugs Aging 2011;28:283–93.
38. Warden V, Hurley AC, Volicer L. Development and psychometric evaluation of the pain assessment in advanced dementia (PAINAD) scale. J Am Med Dir Assoc 2003;4(1):9–15.
39. Romem A, Tom SE, Beauchene M, et al. Pain management at the end of life: a comparative study of cancer, dementia, and chronic obstructive pulmonary disease patients. Palliat Med 2015;29(5):464–9.

40. Hendriks SA, Smalbrugge M, Galindo-Garre F, et al. 6JT. From admission to death: prevalence and course of pain, agitation, and shortness of breath, and treatment of these symptoms in nursing home residents with dementia. J Am Med Dir Assoc 2015;16:475–81.
41. Emmerzaal TL, Kiliaan AJ, Gustafson DR. 2003-2013: a decade of body mass index, Alzheimer's disease, and dementia. J Alzheimers Dis 2015;43:739–55.
42. McGuire MJ, Ishii M. Leptin dysfunction and Alzheimer's disease: evidence from cellular, animal, and human studies. Cell Mol Neurobiol 2016;2:203–17.
43. Morley JE, Thomas DR, Wilson MM. Cachexia: pathophysiology and clinical relevance. Am J Clin Nutr 2006;83:735–43.
44. Palecek EJ, Teno JM, Casarett DJ, et al. Comfort feeding only: a proposal to bring clarity to decision-making regarding difficulty with eating for persons with advanced dementia. J Am Geriatr Soc 2010;58:580–4.
45. Stewart JT, Gorelik AR. Involuntary weight loss associated with cholinesterase inhibitors in dementia. J Am Geriatr Soc 2006;54:1013–4.
46. Ali S, Garcia JM. Sarcopenia, cachexia and aging: diagnosis, mechanisms and therapeutic options - a mini-review. Gerontology 2014;60:294–305.
47. Abu RA, Khoury T, Cohen J, et al. PEG insertion in patients with dementia does not improve nutritional status and has worse outcomes as compared with PEG insertion for other indications. J Clin Gastroenterol 2016. [Epub ahead of print].
48. Mitchell SL, Mor V, Gozalo PL, et al. Tube feeding in US nursing home residents with advanced dementia, 2000-2014. JAMA 2016;316:769–70.
49. Gillick MR, Volandes AE. The standard of caring: why do we still use feeding tubes in patients with advanced dementia? J Am Med Dir Assoc 2008;9:364–7.

Integrated Care for Older Adults with Serious Mental Illness and Medical Comorbidity

Evidence-Based Models and Future Research Directions

Stephen J. Bartels, MD, MS[a],*, Peter R. DiMilia, MPH[b],
Karen L. Fortuna, PhD[c], John A. Naslund, PhD, MPH[d]

KEYWORDS

- Serious mental illness • Older adult • Elderly • Comorbidity • Integrated care
- Collaborative care • Illness self-management

KEY POINTS

- Older adults with serious mental illness have an increased risk of early mortality, medical comorbidity, early institutionalization, and high medical costs.
- Psychosocial skills training, integrated illness self-management, and collaborative care and behavioral health homes are current, evidence-based approaches to integrated care models for older adults with serious mental illness.
- Highly promising integrated care models of the future that incorporate novel uses of telehealth, mobile health technology and peer support, and strategies from developing economies are discussed.

The aging of the baby boomer population is resulting in an unprecedented growth in the number of middle-aged and older adults with serious mental illness (SMI) in the United States. People with SMIs (schizophrenia, schizoaffective disorder, bipolar disorder, and treatment refractory depression) make up to 4% to 6% of the population[1] and experience high rates of comorbid chronic health conditions, with major consequences on life expectancy, functioning, community tenure, and health care costs.

Disclosure Statement: The authors have nothing to disclose.
[a] Dartmouth Centers for Health and Aging, 46 Centerra Parkway, Box 201, Lebanon, NH 03766, USA; [b] The Dartmouth Institute for Health Policy and Clinical Practice, 46 Centerra Parkway, Box 201, Lebanon, NH 03766, USA; [c] Psychiatry, Geisel School of Medicine at Dartmouth, 46 Centerra Parkway, Box 201, Lebanon, NH 03766, USA; [d] Dartmouth Center for Technology and Behavioral Health, 46 Centerra Parkway, Box 201, Lebanon, NH 03766, USA
* Corresponding author.
E-mail address: Stephen.j.bartels@dartmouth.edu

Psychiatr Clin N Am 41 (2018) 153–164
https://doi.org/10.1016/j.psc.2017.10.012
0193-953X/18/© 2017 Elsevier Inc. All rights reserved.

Adults 55 to 64 years old with SMIs are 4 times more likely to die compared with adults without mental illness[2] and are faced with a reduced life expectancy of 11 years to 30 years compared with the general population.[3,4] According to a national sample of Medicaid beneficiaries with schizophrenia (ages 20–64 years old), cardiovascular disease is the most common cause of early mortality.[2] Additional major causes of this early mortality health disparity are largely due to high rates of diabetes, chronic obstructive pulmonary disease, obesity, and tobacco use[5] as well as unrecognized medical disease.[6] Furthermore, as persons with SMIs age, they struggle to maintain community tenure and are 3.5-times more likely to reside in a nursing home compared with other Medicaid beneficiaries of the same age.[7]

Middle-aged to older adults with SMIs have special needs that potentially impede community tenure compared with similarly aged adults without SMIs, including a greater likelihood of impaired independent living skills, inadequate social skills, minimal social support networks, and limited medical and psychiatric self-management skills.[8] The adverse consequences of these needs result in excess medical hospitalizations and premature nursing home placement,[4,7] despite a majority of older adults with SMIs preferring to live in community-based settings.[9] Greater use of acute hospital and nursing homes by older adults with SMIs is largely responsible for health care costs that are 2-times to 3-times greater than those for dually eligible (Medicaid and Medicare) beneficiaries without a mental health condition.[10]

Despite higher acute-care and long-term care costs, SMIs are associated with inadequate, highly variable medical monitoring and treatment[11] and numerous barriers to preventive and routine health care. Half of persons with a psychiatric disorder (59%) report at least 1 barrier to health care, compared with 19% of persons without a mental illness.[12] The greater risk and incidence of adverse outcomes[13] associated with SMIs and medical comorbidity call for innovative models of integrated health care that address high rates of chronic health conditions in this high-risk group.[14–16] The excess risk of early mortality, medical comorbidity, early institutionalization, and disproportionately high costs among persons with SMIs make this group a major priority for developing and disseminating effective and sustainable integrated care models.

The purpose of this overview is to provide a summary of current evidence-based integrated models of care and to identify future promising approaches that address both the mental and physical health needs of older adults with SMIs. Current evidence-based approaches include (1) psychosocial skills training, (2) illness self-management, and (3) collaborative care and behavioral health homes. Finally, a brief overview is provided of highly promising future models that build on these approaches by incorporating novel uses of telehealth and mobile health technology, peer support, and adapting models from developing economies to address under-resourced and unmet needs.

PSYCHOSOCIAL SKILLS TRAINING

This section provides a brief overview of 3 skills training programs specifically designed for older adults with SMIs that proved effective in randomized clinical trials: Helping Older People Experience Success (HOPES); Functional Adaptation Skills Training (FAST); and Cognitive-Behavioral Social Skills Training (CBSST).

Helping Older People Experience Success

HOPES integrates psychosocial skills training and preventive health care management with the goal of enhancing independent functioning and community tenure in older adults with SMIs.[16] The skills training component of HOPES includes classes, role-play exercises, and community-based homework assignments in social skills, community living skills, and healthy living. The weekly co-led skills class curriculum provided over 12 months consists of 7 modules: Communicating Effectively, Making and Keeping Friends, Making the Most of Leisure Time, Healthy Living, Using Medications Effectively, Living Independently in the Community, and Making the Most of a Health Care Visit. Each module includes 6 to 8 component skills and 1 skill is taught each week. The integrated health management component of HOPES begins with a medical history and evaluation of health care needs, including preventive health care, and is delivered by a registered nurse (RN). The RN and participants then collaboratively set health-related goals for managing chronic medical conditions and obtaining recommended preventive care. A randomized controlled trial of HOPES consisting of 183 enrolled older adults (mean age 60 years) with SMIs (28% schizophrenia, 28% schizoaffective disorder, and 24% depression) resulted in improved skills performance, psychosocial functioning, self-efficacy, and psychiatric symptoms at 1-year and 3-year follow-ups compared with usual care.[17] In addition, compared with the usual care group, a greater proportion of HOPES participants received blood pressure screening, flu shots, hearing tests, eye examinations, visual acuity tests, mammograms, and Papanicolaou smears and nearly twice as many completed advanced directives.

Functional Adaptation Skills Training

FAST is a psychosocial intervention for community-dwelling middle-aged and older adults with schizophrenia spectrum disorder or psychotic mood disorders.[18] Based on social-cognitive theory and Liberman and Colleagues' Social and Independent Living Skills Program,[19] FAST provides group sessions aimed at improving 6 everyday skills: medication management, social skills, communication skills, organization and planning, transportation, and financial management in 4, 120-minute group sessions over the course of 24 weeks. Active learning approaches are used that include in-session skills practice, behavioral modeling, role-playing, reinforcement, and homework practice assignments. A randomized controlled trial of the FAST program was conducted by Patterson and colleagues,[18] including 240 older adults (greater than 40 years old, mean participant age 51 years old) with schizophrenia (80.6%) or schizoaffective disorder (19.4%) from 25 board and care facilities. Compared with participants in the control condition, FAST program participants showed significantly improved everyday functional skills on the University of California, San Diego, Performance-based Skills Assessment and social and communication skills on the Social Skills Performance Assessment after 6 months. FAST program participants were approximately 60% less likely than the control group to use emergency medical services throughout the 6-month intervention, although emergency service use did not differ between FAST and control participants at 1-year postintervention (18 months from baseline). Building on these findings, FAST has been adapted for monolingual Spanish-speaking, middle-aged, and older Latino adults with schizophrenia.[20] A pilot study of the adapted version of the FAST program, Programa de Entrenamiento para el Desarrollo de Aptitudes para Latinos, reported encouraging results with improved functioning and well-being in middle-aged to older Latinos with persistent psychotic illness.[20]

Cognitive-Behavioral Social Skills Training

CBSST is a group therapy program designed to help middle-aged and older adults with schizophrenia attain personalized functioning goals. CBSST combines properties of cognitive-behavioral therapy and social skills training within the framework of the biopsychosocial stress-vulnerability model of schizophrenia.[21] CBSST incorporates self-management, conversation skills, and interpersonal problem-solving techniques to enhance self-efficacy of and improve community tenure for older adults with schizophrenia. This integrated treatment program consists of 3 modules, each delivered over 4 weekly, 2-hour group therapy sessions (12 total sessions). Skills include promoting cognitive-behavioral strategies, recognition of early warning signs of relapse, improved communication with health care professionals and social interactions in everyday activities, treatment adherence, and behavioral strategies for coping with symptoms of mental illness.[22] Weekly homework exercises are assigned to participants to reinforce skills learned during the group therapy session. A randomized controlled trial compared CBSST with treatment as usual among a cohort of community-dwelling, middle-aged to older adults (greater than 40 years old, mean participant age 54 years old) with schizophrenia or schizoaffective disorder. At the end of the 6-month intervention, participants in CBSST, compared with the control condition, demonstrated greater engagement in social functioning activities, cognitive insight, and skills. After a 12-month follow-up, CBSST participants reported significantly greater social functioning and comprehension of CBSST skills.[22]

The 3 models evaluated in these studies include several common components. First, all are group-based, as opposed to individually focused, which supports the feasibility and practical application of group-based interventions in older adults with SMIs. Second, these interventions provide accommodations for individuals with physical or cognitive disabilities and develop skills in incremental steps. Finally, these interventions use age-appropriate cognitive-behavioral principles and skills training techniques to meet the specific needs of older persons. Based on the outcomes reported in these studies, social skills training has been demonstrated to be feasible and associated with improvement in key dimensions of social functioning and independent community living for older adults with SMIs.[23]

ILLNESS SELF-MANAGEMENT

Traditionally, illness self-management programs have addressed either chronic physical health or mental health conditions but not both. In contrast, integrated medical and psychiatric self-management programs combine self-management of both physical and mental health disorders.[24] A recent systematic review identified 3 interventions targeting self-management of chronic health conditions for persons with SMIs: the Health and Recovery Peer (HARP) program, Targeted Training in Illness Management (TTIM), and Integrated Illness Management and Recovery (I-IMR).[25]

Health and Recovery Peer Program

The HARP program[26] is an illness self-management intervention adapted from the Chronic Disease Self-Management Program[27] for adults with SMIs. The HARP program consists of 6 peer specialist-led sessions covering topics including illness self-management, exercise and physical activity, pain and fatigue management, healthy eating with a limited budget, medication management, and finding and working with a consistent physician. The peer specialists also encourage participants to set short-term goals for health behavior change through identification of negative health behavior and potential manageable ways to improve. The potential effectiveness of HARP was evaluated in a randomized controlled pilot study in a community mental health center[26] in 80 adults (mean age 48 years) with SMIs (schizophrenia 29% and bipolar disorder 33%) and comorbid, chronic physical health conditions (hypertension 63%, arthritis 50%, and heart disease 23%). At the end of a 6-month follow-up, HARP program participants, compared with the usual care group, reported significantly greater perceived ability to manage their own illnesses, better medication adherence, better health-related quality of life, and greater use of primary care.[26]

Targeted Training in Illness Management

TTIM is a group-based, peer-facilitated, illness self-management program for community-dwelling adults with SMIs and comorbid diabetes mellitus.[28] Drawing from both the Life Goals Program and the Diabetes Awareness and Rehabilitation Training models, the TTIM program blends mental health and diabetes care with social support from peer educators to deliver an illness self-management program, including psychoeducation, problem identification, goal setting, behavioral modeling, and care coordination. In the first phase of TTIM, participants engage in 12 weekly group sessions consisting of 6 to 10 participants, the nurse educator, and the peer specialist covering topics, such as medication management, nutrition, exercise, substance use, problem-solving skills, engaging social support systems, and setting personal goals. In the second phase of TTIM, the nurse educator and peer specialist engage participants in brief maintenance sessions over the telephone. In a randomized controlled trial of 200 adults (mean age 53 years) with SMIs (schizophrenia 25% and major depressive disorder 48%) and diabetes mellitus, TTIM program participants reported improved psychiatric symptoms and general functioning compared with usual care.[28] TTIM participants demonstrated significantly greater knowledge of diabetes compared with the control group and 98% of TTIM participants considered the program to be useful. No differences were found, however, between the intervention and control groups with respect to general health status, self-management of diabetes, systolic blood pressure, or body mass index.

Integrated Illness Management and Recovery

I-IMR is a recovery-oriented intervention that combines training and coaching in both psychiatric and medical illness self-management into a single integrated curriculum and program aimed at improving outcomes for older adults (ages 50 and older) with SMIs and chronic health conditions.[29,30] I-IMR was developed by adding medical illness self-management training[27] to the evidence-based practice of mental illness management and recovery, consisting of psychoeducation, behavioral tailoring, training in relapse prevention, and cognitive-behavioral techniques.[31] For each psychiatric self-management skill module, there is a corresponding medical illness self-management training component, including modules on recovery and wellness, common mental and physical health conditions, stress vulnerability, social supports, medication adherence, relapse prevention, coping with stress, coping with symptoms of mental and physical distress, substance and medication misuse, and navigating mental health and medical health care delivery systems. In I-IMR, skills training is provided by a specialist guided by modules complemented by health care management provided by a nurse or health outreach worker. I-IMR combines 4 evidence-based psychosocial interventions shown effective among people with SMIs: (1) psychoeducation, which improves knowledge about mental illness management; (2) behavioral tailoring, which improves medication adherence; (3) relapse prevention training, which decreases relapses and rehospitalizations; and (4) coping skills training, which reduces distress related to symptoms. In a randomized study comparing I-IMR (n = 36) to usual care (n = 35), I-IMR was associated with improved psychiatric illness self-management, improved diabetes self-management, and decreased hospitalizations.[30]

In summary, despite the common occurrence of both psychiatric and medical illness in older adults with SMIs, there remains a paucity of integrated medical and psychiatric self-management programs that combine self-management of both physical and mental health disorders. HARP and TTIM primarily focus on medical illness self-management interventions for persons with SMIs and include all ages. In contrast, I-IMR provides a balanced curriculum of both psychiatric and medical self-management and is specifically designed for older adults.[25]

COLLABORATIVE CARE AND BEHAVIORAL HEALTH HOMES

More than 15 years ago, 3 concurrent multisite randomized trials evaluated the effectiveness of integrating mental health in primary care for older adults: Primary Care Research in Substance Abuse and Mental Health for the Elderly (funded by the Substance Abuse and Mental Health Services Administration),[32] Prevention of Suicide in Primary Care Elderly: Collaborative Trial (funded by the National Institute of Mental Health),[33] and Improving Mood—Promoting Access to Collaborative Treatment (funded by the John A. Hartford Foundation).[34] This unprecedented convergence of research on older adults with mental health conditions in primary care established the evidence base for integrating mental health into primary care settings as superior to specialty referral in engaging older adults in mental health and substance use disorder treatment,[32] while also establishing integrated collaborative care as superior to usual care in managing depression.[33,34] An extensive research literature now documents the effectiveness of the collaborative care model for mental health conditions.[35]

In contrast to extensive research focused on embedding mental health in primary care, remarkably little research has studied embedding primary care within mental health service delivery settings. Based on the concept of the patient-centered medical home, behavioral health homes have been proposed as a promising approach to address the challenges of persons with SMIs with chronic health conditions by providing integrated delivery of primary health care. In a review of the extent literature, the authors identified 3 randomized control trials of behavioral health homes that focused on adults ages 18 years and older with SMIs and comorbid medical conditions.

An early randomized controlled pilot study compared an integrated care model to usual care (ie, referral to Veterans Affairs general medicine clinic) in a sample of 120 veterans with SMIs (mean age 45.7).[36] Primary care services were co-located in Veterans Affairs mental health clinics and staffed by primary care providers and a nurse case manager. Primary care providers coordinated care and communicated regularly with staff at mental health clinics and emphasized patient education and preventive health services. After 12 months, patients treated at the integrated care clinic had more primary care visits, received more preventive services, and experienced a greater improvement on the physical component of the 36-Item Short Form Health Survey (SF-36) (4.7 points vs −0.3 points) compared with usual care.[36]

A subsequent randomized controlled trial of 407 adults with SMIs (mean age 47) compared a behavioral health home model (Primary Care Access, Referral, and Evaluation [PCARE]) to usual care (ie, usual care participants were provided with a list of contact information to independently contact local primary care medical clinics).[37] PCARE included 2 full-time nurse care managers who coordinate care for patients between behavioral health and medical providers. The care managers used motivational interviewing to enhance patient activation, promote self-management skills and health advocacy skills, and develop action plans to support health behavior change. After 12 months, the PCARE intervention group demonstrated significantly more primary care service use, greater improvement on the SF-36 mental component, and clinically significant reduction in Framingham Risk Score for 10-year cardiovascular risk compared with the usual care group.

Finally, a third randomized controlled trial with 447 adults with SMIs (mean age 47.3) compared outcomes for participants in the Substance Abuse and Mental Health Services Administration's Primary and Behavioral Health Care Integration (PBHCI) program with usual care.[38] Compared with usual care, the PBHCI behavioral health home was associated with significantly greater use of preventive services, quality of cardiometabolic care, and continuity of care. Although systolic blood pressure showed a greater reduction in the behavioral health home model compared with usual care (1.8 points), this was not clinically significant and no differences were found in diastolic blood pressure, total cholesterol and low-density lipoprotein cholesterol, blood glucose, hemoglobin A_{1c}, patient activation, or the Framingham Risk Score.

In summary, integrated health homes have the potential to significantly increase the quality and amount of preventive services offered to persons with SMIs, but inconsistently achieve clinically significant results. Improved outcomes for patients with SMIs enrolled in behavioral health homes, however, are more likely with the addition of self-management techniques to enhance patient involvement in care and attention to physical health.[37–40]

FUTURE DIRECTIONS
Automated Telehealth and Mobile Health

Advances in health technology offer a highly promising alternative approach to illness self-management for people with chronic health conditions.[41] Automated telehealth interventions have been developed to improve the daily management of chronic health conditions by providing in-home prompting of adherence to prescribed treatment and remote monitoring of symptoms, including biometric measures. Predetermined algorithms have the capacity to determine trends in key indicators to identify individuals who are most at risk of hospitalization, triggering early preemptive nurse interventions. In a 6-month study of 70 participants with SMIs and chronic health conditions, investigators at Dartmouth Centers for Health and Aging demonstrated that an automated telehealth intervention has the potential to achieve highly promising results with respect to adherence, self-efficacy, and clinically significant improvements in key chronic health conditions in persons with SMIs. In this pilot study, 89% of participants engaged in 70% or more of the telehealth sessions and 83% rated their ability to manage their medical condition as "much better" postintervention. Participants experienced significant improvements in self-efficacy for managing depression and diastolic blood pressure. The intervention was especially effective for the 67% of participants with SMIs and co-occurring diabetes, who experienced a mean decrease in fasting glucose from baseline (139 mg/dL) to 6 months (113 mg/dL) as well as a significant decrease in urgent care health visits.[42]

In addition to automated telehealth programs, mobile and online technologies (eg, smartphone applications and social media) have the potential to improve self-management and delivery of interventions to adults with SMIs.[43] For example, mobile and online technologies allow for the standardization of delivering evidence-based intervention components, have the capacity to repeat intervention modules any time or in any place, offer on-demand access to live or automated support, have the ability to be automatically customized to patients' preferences and recovery goals, and have the capacity to simultaneously address multiple psychiatric and medical conditions.[44]

Peer Support, Technology, and Social Media

The combination of certified peer specialists and technology in the delivery of integrated self-management interventions has the potential to accelerate the adoption of technology-based interventions.[45] In an effort to leverage the potential of technology and peer-supported delivery, I-IMR[30] has been adapted to be delivered by a certified peer specialist facilitated by automated e-modules, a smartphone application, and a peer care management dashboard (PeerTECH).[44,46] The preliminary feasibility of PeerTECH has been established in a pilot study for older adults with SMIs. Using a pre–post design, 8 adults ages 60 years and older with SMIs and medical comorbidity (ie, cardiovascular disease, obesity, or diabetes) received PeerTECH in their homes over a 12-week period. Participants completed more than 70% of daily self-management tasks on the smartphone application and reported improved psychiatric illness self-management and medical self-management, hope, empowerment, and quality of life.[47] This promising evidence suggests that the innovative use of peers and technology potentially offers the capacity to increase the dose of the intervention without additional in-person sessions, potentially reducing staff time and efforts, duration, and downstream costs.

Several recent studies have also documented the increasing access and use of social media among adults with SMIs. For example, in a survey of individuals with SMIs receiving community mental health services, these individuals reported comparable rates of Facebook and Twitter use as the general population.[48] Other studies have found that many people with SMIs are turning to social media to share their personal experiences of living with a mental illness, to seek mental health information and advice, to learn from others, or to provide support to other individuals facing similar challenging mental health problems.[49] A recent survey found that people with SMIs expressed interest in receiving services for both their mental and physical health concerns delivered using popular social media.[50] As social media continues to become an important part of the daily lives of many individuals living with SMIs,[49] there may be ways to use social media to support collaborative care. For example, social media integrated within a collaborative care model could potentially allow older adults with SMIs to connect with others who share similar mental and physical health concerns and seek support and advice from a community of peers.[49]

Reverse Innovation: Adapting Potential Solutions from Low-Income and Middle-Income Countries

Addressing the future shortfall in geriatric mental health services will require new models of care, including novel workforce solutions, such as community health workers, lay and peer-based outreach services, and use of telehealth and mobile technology.[51] Reverse innovation is a concept that describes adapting innovative approaches developed in low-income and middle-income countries to help solve under-resourced challenges in developed economies.[52] Preliminary studies highlight older adults' increasing access to mobile devices as well as early efforts using technology to support chronic medical care in the elderly. In a sample of 559 primary care patients in La Paz, Bolivia, approximately half screened positive for depression, 58% were age 50 and older, and 86% reported owning a mobile phone.[53] Remarkably, more than 71% of respondents ages 65 and older owned a mobile phone.[53] In a survey of 201 people with SMIs from Rajasthan, India, approximately 30% of respondents were ages 50 and older, more than 70% had access to a mobile phone, and more than 80% expressed an interest in receiving mental health services by phone.[54] Mobile technologies have also been used to facilitate monitoring and management of chronic medical conditions among the elderly in China.[55] In response to aging populations in Latin America, there are currently multinational efforts spanning Brazil and Peru aimed at leveraging digital technology to address co-occurring depression and diabetes within primary care settings.[56] Additional opportunities include using digital technology to enhance existing community-based depression care programs for older adults[57] or to help with raising awareness about mental disorders in late life, engaging family supports, and coordinating training in geriatric mental health care among community health workers.[58]

SUMMARY

In contrast to a large number of evidence-based practices for older adults with depression and other common mental health conditions, a limited array of interventions has been developed and empirically evaluated for older adults (ages 50 and older) with SMIs (schizophrenia, schizoaffective disorder, bipolar disorder, and treatment refractory depression). The co-occurrence of chronic medical conditions in this population has resulted in a small array of interventions aimed at addressing both mental health and physical health conditions in this rapidly growing, complex population at high risk for hospital and nursing home care and early mortality. Effective future strategies for addressing this high-cost, high-risk emerging population will require new models of community-based intervention and rehabilitation that combine mental health and physical health care, assisted by technology and new models of health outreach and support.

REFERENCES

1. Kessler RC, Chiu WT, Demler O, et al. Prevalence, severity, and comorbidity of 12-month DSM-IV disorders in the National Comorbidity Survey Replication. Arch Gen Psychiatry 2005;62(6):617–27.
2. Olfson M, Gerhard T, Huang C, et al. Premature mortality among adults with schizophrenia in the United States. JAMA Psychiatry 2015;72(12):1172–81.
3. Walker ER, McGee RE, Druss BG. Mortality in mental disorders and global disease burden implications: a systematic review and meta-analysis. JAMA Psychiatry 2015;72(4):334–41.
4. Druss BG, Zhao L, Von Esenwein S, et al. Understanding excess mortality in persons with mental illness: 17-year follow up of a nationally representative US survey. Med Care 2011;49(6):599–604.
5. DE Hert M, Correll CU, Bobes J, et al. Physical illness in patients with severe mental disorders. I. Prevalence, impact of medications and disparities in health care. World Psychiatry 2011;10(1):52–77.
6. Jeste DV, Gladsjo JA, Lindamer LA, et al. Medical comorbidity in schizophrenia. Schizophr Bull 1996;22(3):413–30.
7. Andrews AO, Bartels SJ, Xie H, et al. Increased risk of nursing home admission among middle aged and older adults with schizophrenia. Am J Geriatr Psychiatry 2009;17(8):697–705.
8. Druss BG, Bradford DW, Rosenheck RA, et al. Mental disorders and use of cardiovascular procedures after myocardial infarction. JAMA 2000;283(4):506–11.
9. Horan ME, Muller JJ, Winocur S, et al. Quality of life in boarding houses and hostels: a residents' perspective. Community Ment Health J 2001;37(4):323–34.
10. Bartels SJ, Clark RE, Peacock WJ, et al. Medicare and medicaid costs for schizophrenia patients by age cohort compared with costs for depression, dementia, and medically ill patients. Am J Geriatr Psychiatry 2003;11(6):648–57.
11. Druss BG, Rosenheck RA, Desai MM, et al. Quality of preventive medical care for patients with mental disorders. Med Care 2002;40(2):129–36.

12. Dickerson FB, McNary SW, Brown CH, et al. Somatic healthcare utilization among adults with serious mental illness who are receiving community psychiatric services. Med Care 2003;41(4):560–70.

13. Viron MJ, Stern TA. The impact of serious mental illness on health and healthcare. Psychosomatics 2010;51(6):458–65.

14. Bartels SJ. Caring for the whole person: integrated health care for older adults with severe mental illness and medical comorbidity. J Am Geriatr Soc 2004; 52(12 Suppl):S249–57.

15. Bartels SJ, Forester B, Mueser KT, et al. Enhanced skills training and health care management for older persons with severe mental illness. Community Ment Health J 2004;40(1):75–90.

16. Pratt SI, Bartels SJ, Mueser KT, et al. Helping older people experience success: an integrated model of psychosocial rehabilitation and health care management for older adults with serious mental illness. Am J Psychiatr Rehabil 2008;11(1): 41–60.

17. Bartels SJ, Pratt SI, Mueser KT, et al. Long-term outcomes of a randomized trial of integrated skills training and preventive healthcare for older adults with serious mental illness. Am J Geriatr Psychiatry 2014;22(11):1251–61.

18. Patterson TL, Mausbach BT, McKibbin C, et al. Functional adaptation skills training (FAST): a randomized trial of a psychosocial intervention for middle-aged and older patients with chronic psychotic disorders. Schizophr Res 2006; 86(1–3):291–9.

19. Psychiatric Rehabilitation Consultants. Modules in the UCLA Social and Independent Living Skill Series. Camarillo (CA): Psychiatric Rehabilitation Consultants; 1991.

20. Mausbach BT, Bucardo J, Cardenas V, et al. Evaluation of a culturally tailored skills intervention for latinos with persistent psychotic disorders. Am J Psychiatr Rehabil 2008;11(1):61–75.

21. McQuaid JR, Granholm E, McClure FS, et al. Development of an integrated cognitive-behavioral and social skills training intervention for older patients with schizophrenia. J Psychother Pract Res 2000;9(3):149–56.

22. Granholm E, McQuaid JR, McClure FS, et al. A randomized, controlled trial of cognitive behavioral social skills training for middle-aged and older outpatients with chronic schizophrenia. Am J Psychiatry 2005;162(3):520–9.

23. Pratt SI, Van Citters AD, Mueser KT, et al. Psychosocial rehabilitation in older adults with serious mental illness: a review of the research literature and recommendations for development of rehabilitative approaches. Am J Psychiatr Rehabil 2008;11(1):7–40.

24. Corbin JM, Strauss AL. Unending work and care: managing chronic illness at home. San Francisco (CA): Jossey-Bass; 1988.

25. Whiteman KL, Naslund JA, DiNapoli EA, et al. Systematic review of integrated general medical and psychiatric self-management interventions for adults with serious mental illness. Psychiatr Serv 2016;67(11):1213–25.

26. Druss BG, Zhao L, von Esenwein SA, et al. The Health and Recovery Peer (HARP) Program: a peer-led intervention to improve medical self-management for persons with serious mental illness. Schizophr Res 2010;118(1–3):264–70.

27. Lorig KR, Sobel DS, Stewart AL, et al. Evidence suggesting that a chronic disease self-management program can improve health status while reducing hospitalization - A randomized trial. Med Care 1999;37(1):5–14.

28. Sajatovic M, Gunzler DD, Kanuch SW, et al. A 60-Week Prospective RCT of a Self-Management Intervention for Individuals With Serious Mental Illness and Diabetes Mellitus. Psychiatr Serv 2017;68(9):883–90.
29. Mueser KT, Bartels SJ, Santos M, et al. Integrated illness management and recovery: a program for integrating physical and psychiatric illness self-management in older persons with severe mental illness. Am J Psychiatr Rehabil 2012;15(2): 131–56.
30. Bartels SJ, Pratt SI, Mueser KT, et al. Integrated IMR for psychiatric and general medical illness for adults aged 50 or older with serious mental illness. Psychiatr Serv 2014;65(3):330–7.
31. Mueser KT, Corrigan PW, Hilton DW, et al. Illness management and recovery: a review of the research. Psychiatr Serv 2002;53(10):1272–84.
32. Bartels SJ, Coakley EH, Zubritsky C, et al. Improving access to geriatric mental health services: a randomized trial comparing treatment engagement with integrated versus enhanced referral care for depression, anxiety, and at-risk alcohol use. Am J Psychiatry 2004;161(8):1455–62.
33. Bruce ML, Ten Have TR, Reynolds CF 3rd, et al. Reducing suicidal ideation and depressive symptoms in depressed older primary care patients: a randomized controlled trial. JAMA 2004;291(9):1081–91.
34. Unutzer J, Katon W, Callahan CM, et al. Collaborative care management of late-life depression in the primary care setting: a randomized controlled trial. JAMA 2002;288(22):2836–45.
35. Woltmann E, Grogan-Kaylor A, Perron B, et al. Comparative effectiveness of collaborative chronic care models for mental health conditions across primary, specialty, and behavioral health care settings: systematic review and meta-analysis. Am J Psychiatry 2012;169(8):790–804.
36. Druss BG, Rohrbaugh RM, Levinson CM, et al. Integrated medical care for patients with serious psychiatric illness: a randomized trial. Arch Gen Psychiatry 2001;58(9):861–8.
37. Druss BG, von Esenwein SA, Compton MT, et al. A randomized trial of medical care management for community mental health settings: the primary care access, referral, and evaluation (PCARE) study. Am J Psychiatry 2010;167(2): 151–9.
38. Druss BG, von Esenwein SA, Glick GE, et al. Randomized Trial of an integrated behavioral health home: the health outcomes management and evaluation (HOME) study. Am J Psychiatry 2017;174(3):246–55.
39. Gilmer TP, Henwood BF, Goode M, et al. Implementation of Integrated health homes and health outcomes for persons with serious mental illness in Los Angeles county. Psychiatr Serv 2016;67(10):1062–7.
40. Bartels SJ, Aschbrenner KA, Rolin SA, et al. Activating older adults with serious mental illness for collaborative primary care visits. Psychiatr Rehabil J 2013;36(4): 278–88.
41. Godleski L, Cervone D, Vogel D, et al. Home telemental health implementation and outcomes using electronic messaging. J Telemed Telecare 2012;18(1):17–9.
42. Pratt SI, Bartels SJ, Mueser KT, et al. Feasibility and effectiveness of an automated telehealth intervention to improve illness self-management in people with serious psychiatric and medical disorders. Psychiatr Rehabil J 2013;36(4): 297–305.
43. Naslund JA, Marsch LA, McHugo GJ, et al. Emerging mHealth and eHealth interventions for serious mental illness: a review of the literature. J Ment Health 2015; 24(5):321–32.

44. Whiteman KL, Lohman MC, Bartels SJ. A peer- and technology-supported self-management intervention. Psychiatr Serv 2017;68(4):420.

45. Mohr DC, Cuijpers P, Lehman K. Supportive accountability: a model for providing human support to enhance adherence to eHealth interventions. J Med Internet Res 2011;13(1):e30.

46. Whiteman KL, Lohman MC, Gill LE, et al. Adapting a psychosocial intervention for smartphone delivery to middle-aged and older adults with serious mental illness. Am J Geriatr Psychiatry 2017;25(8):819–28.

47. Fortuna KL, DiMilia PR, Lohman MC, et al. Feasibility, aceptability, and preliminary effectiveness of a peer-delivered and technology supported self-management intervention for older adults with serious mental illness. Psychiatr Q 2017. [Epub ahead of print].

48. Naslund JA, Aschbrenner KA, Bartels SJ. How people living with serious mental illness use smartphones, mobile apps, and social media. Psychiatr Rehabil J 2016;39(4):364–7.

49. Naslund JA, Aschbrenner KA, Marsch LA, et al. The future of mental health care: peer-to-peer support and social media. Epidemiol Psychiatr Sci 2016;25(2):113–22.

50. Naslund JA, Aschbrenner KA, McHugo GJ, et al. Exploring opportunities to support mental health care using social media: a survey of social media users with mental illness. Early Interv Psychiatry 2017. [Epub ahead of print].

51. Bartels SJ, Naslund JA. The underside of the silver tsunami—older adults and mental health care. N Engl J Med 2013;368(6):493–6.

52. Govindarajan V, Trimble C. Reverse innovation: create far from home, win everywhere. Boston: Harvard Business School Publishing; 2012.

53. Kamis K, Janevic MR, Marinec N, et al. A study of mobile phone use among patients with noncommunicable diseases in La Paz, Bolivia: implications for mHealth research and development. Global Health 2015;11(1):1.

54. Jain N, Singh H, Koolwal GD, et al. Opportunities and barriers in service delivery through mobile phones (mHealth) for severe mental illnesses in Rajasthan, India: a multi-site study. Asian J Psychiatr 2015;14:31–5.

55. Lv Z, Xia F, Wu G, et al. iCare: a mobile health monitoring system for the elderly. Paper presented at: Proceedings of the 2010 IEEE/ACM Int'l Conference on Green Computing and Communications & Int'l Conference on Cyber, Physical and Social Computing. Hangzhou, China. December 18–20, 2010.

56. Bonini B, Araya R, Quayle J, et al. LATIN-MH: a model for building research capacity within Latin America. Glob Ment Health (Camb) 2017;4:e2.

57. Chen S, Conwell Y, He J, et al. Depression care management for adults older than 60 years in primary care clinics in urban China: a cluster-randomised trial. Lancet Psychiatry 2015;2(4):332–9.

58. Patel V, Prince M. Ageing and mental health in a developing country: who cares? Qualitative studies from Goa, India. Psychol Med 2001;31(01):29–38.

Posttraumatic Stress Disorder in the Elderly

Rebekah J. Jakel, MD, PhD*

KEYWORDS

- Posttraumatic stress disorder • PTSD • Elderly • Aging • Dementia • Trauma

KEY POINTS

- Posttraumatic stress disorder (PTSD) can arise from a variety of different traumatic stressors and can have long-lasting impact.
- Chronic PTSD is associated with poorer health outcomes, including cardiovascular disease and dementia as compared to those without PTSD.
- Older adults should receive treatment of PTSD with attention to age-related changes in drug metabolism and comorbidities.

Exposure to traumatic events can occur across the life span. Although most people respond to trauma with some level of psychological distress, most return to pretrauma levels of health within 3 months. A subset continues to have persistent and debilitating cognitive, behavioral, arousal symptoms as part of posttraumatic stress disorder (PTSD) that may resolve or become chronic. The *Diagnostic and Statistical Manual of Mental Disorders* (Fifth Edition)[1] defines exposure to actual or threatened trauma as direct, witnessed as occurring in others, learning of violent events that occurred to a close family member, or repeated exposure to details of trauma. Symptom clusters include intrusion symptoms of recurrent, distressing memories, nightmares, flashbacks, avoidance of reminders of the trauma, negative cognitions and mood associated with the traumatic events, and hyperarousal symptoms that occur greater than 1 month, cause distress, and have no other known cause.

The lifetime prevalence of PTSD is 8.7% by age 75 using *Diagnostic and Statistical Manual of Mental Disorders* (Fifth Edition) criteria.[1] It has been hypothesized that women are at increased risk of PTSD given recognized increased vulnerability to comorbid mood disorders; however, women may be at increased risk of exposure to traumatic events, especially interpersonal violence, such as sexual and domestic violence. Patients with PTSD are 80% more likely to have comorbid psychiatric disorders,

Disclosure: The author has nothing to disclose.
Department of Psychiatry and Behavioral Sciences, Duke University Medical Center, 3950, Durham, NC 27710, USA
* Durham VA Medical Center, 116A, 508 Fulton Street, Durham, NC 27705.
E-mail address: rebekah.jakel@duke.edu

Psychiatr Clin N Am 41 (2018) 165–175
https://doi.org/10.1016/j.psc.2017.10.013
0193-953X/18/Published by Elsevier Inc.

including mood, anxiety, and substance use disorders.[1] Although not typically considered a disorder of aging, PTSD may differentially affect the geriatric population. The purpose of this article is to review PTSD as it has impacts on aging and the elderly.

It is not clear why some persons develop PTSD and others do not. The nature of the trauma as well as the frequency and severity likely has an impact on the development and course of PTSD. There are many different types of possible traumatic events: natural disasters, human-caused disasters, experiences of war as a civilian or a soldier, and interpersonal violence, such as sexual or physical trauma. The individual experience of "trauma" may differ related to the nature of the trauma as well as an individual's perception of the meaning of the event. The developmental stage at the time of trauma likely also has an impact on the expression of traumatic-based symptoms. Clearly, children of different ages process the same event differently. How this is extrapolated through the life span is unclear, however. The variability of experiences as a function of developmental timing likely accounts for some of the variation of trauma-based pathology, symptomatic expression, and prognosis. The examination of PTSD within the elderly population can include the impact of trauma occurring in early childhood through the twilight years as well as the accumulation of traumatic events throughout the life span. Controlling and accounting for this is a daunting task.

Much of the current understanding of PTSD has been derived from studies of veterans of major conflicts, such as World War II and the Vietnam War. Military experience typically occurs in early adulthood and the cohorts studied have largely been white men. The reliance on retrospective design and focus on specific cohorts may limit the generalizability of the data to other populations.

IMPACT OF ACUTE TRAUMA ON OLDER ADULTS

The impact of acute trauma on the elderly is not well understood and this may reflect the challenge to design studies that control for the multitude of conditions and processes that also correlate with aging, including cumulative trauma. The inoculation hypothesis proposes that exposure to trauma at different points in time is protective, or inoculates against the effects of subsequent traumas with age. Israeli residents exposed to on average 7 years of rocket fire were assessed for trauma-based symptoms using a telephone survey. Older age did correlate with increased symptom burden; however, prior exposure to other traumatic events attenuated this risk.[2] The mechanism of this protection is unknown; it is hypothesized that prior trauma exposure allows for the development of coping strategies that mitigate risks of subsequent trauma and risk of PTSD.

Traumas could also act cumulatively to exacerbate vulnerability to PTSD, perhaps by triggering the memories of older painful events. Aging male veterans (50–65 years) were assessed for psychiatric disorders, combat exposure, and PTSD at 2 time points. Exposure to combat predicted a diagnosis of PTSD, which was associated with increased current level of stress.[3] This suggests that trauma history confers a vulnerability to acute stress and possibly PTSD.

The elderly could be differentially vulnerable to PTSD independent of their prior life traumas. Age-related factors, including worsening cognition, changes in roles (retirement or caregiver roles), losses of family and friends, increasing debility, and changes in health could enhance the pathogenicity of a traumatic event. On the contrary, age may also be associated with resilience and a life perspective that renders older individuals less vulnerable to developing PTSD after traumatic experiences.

It is also possible that advancing age is not a factor in the development of PTSD. A retrospective study of community dwellers exposed to an aircraft crash assessed at

6 months to 7 months after the event via self-report instruments of coping, general health, and impact scales did not demonstrate differential effects in the elderly. Although age did not predict vulnerability to trauma-based symptoms, rates of intrusive thoughts and avoidance correlated with general health problems.[4]

At present, there are not enough data to make conclusions about the differential vulnerability of the elderly to PTSD. This may be due to methodologic challenges, including the ability to control for factors related to both the individuals and trauma. Because subjects are typically identified after trauma, it can be difficult to rate pre-trauma functioning. There is also no uniform way to rate severity of a trauma. Cultural barriers to acknowledging or revealing traumatic experiences may also limit the acquisition of data.

TYPE OF TRAUMATIC EVENT

Much understanding of PTSD in the elderly has come from the study of combat veterans and victims of the Holocaust; however, most PTSD occurs outside the context of combat. It is plausible that characteristics of the inciting traumatic event may also have an impact on the development and prognosis of PTSD in the elderly. Traumatic events can be random and impersonal, such as disasters from natural events, accidents, technological disasters, or acts of terrorism. Interpersonal trauma can occur as sexual or physical violence, within the context of a domestic relationship or by a stranger. The symptomatology of PTSD involves the effects of a trauma on cognition, and the type of trauma may dictate the resultant trauma-based cognitions.[1] A woman may make negative conclusions about herself after an interpersonal trauma that may differ from the self-attributions made after enduring a natural disaster. In fact, women may be more at risk of PTSD than men owing to the high incidence of sexual violence toward women and in domestic violence situations.[5] As women age, their symptoms may be attributed to depression or anxiety, conditions that are also found in women with higher rates of incidence as compared to males, possibly due to failure to screen for remote traumas.[5] Lifetime rates of PTSD may be as high as 20% in American women compared with 8% of men.[6]

Advancing age may increase the risk of exposure to certain types of traumas. Sexual minorities are at elevated risk of interpersonal violence and this risk may be exacerbated with reliance on caregivers. Elderly in residential care may be vulnerable to abuse from other residents or staff.[7] Although not necessarily specific to the elderly, hospitalizations, especially within an ICU setting, have been associated with PTSD. A prospective, observational study of patients ages 60 and older who underwent a noncardiac surgery under general anesthesia showed a rate of 12% having symptoms of PTSD 3 months after surgery. Regression analyses suggested that postoperative delirium was an independent risk factor for PTSD (odds ratio [OR] 2.411; CI, 1.064–5.464), whereas preoperative diagnosis of depression was shown protective.[8]

OUTCOMES ASSOCIATED WITH POSTTRAUMATIC STRESS DISORDER WITH AGING AND IN THE ELDERLY

In addition to the burden of symptoms that constitute PTSD, the elderly may be at risk for further adverse outcomes. PTSD has been associated with increased risk of suicide, changes in physical health and functional performance, and dementia in the elderly. The causal link of these associations is unclear. It is possible that PTSD shares a common underlying pathogenetic mechanism with these adverse outcomes or PTSD could alter health-related behaviors that confer risk for the associated conditions.

Suicide

Although the strongest predictor for suicide is depression, other psychiatric disorders can confer increased risk for suicide. In a retrospective study, elderly patients who attempted suicide admitted to an Israeli psychiatric hospital over a 5-year period were compared with admitted elderly patients without an attempt. Of the eligible patients, 24% of Holocaust survivors had attempted suicide compared with 8.2% of those who were not exposed to the conditions of World War II, suggesting a role for trauma in suicidality.[9] Older male veterans surveyed regarding current suicidal ideation and past attempts revealed that combat veterans were more likely to contemplate suicide (9.2%) than noncombat veterans (4.0%). PTSD was independently associated with suicidality, which was mitigated by social connectedness.[10]

Because PTSD and depression are frequently comorbid conditions, it has been hypothesized that the risk of suicide with PTSD may be explained by comorbid depression. A German study of people ages 60 years to 85 years examined PTSD, depression, and suicidality via rating scales, with suicidal ideation the primary outcome. Suicidal ideation correlated with the number of traumatic experiences with an OR of 1.16 ($P = .011$) compared with those without suicidal ideation. PTSD was diagnosed in 12.4% of subjects with suicidal ideation compared with 3.4% of those who did not meet criteria for PTSD. When depressive symptoms were controlled, the association of suicidal ideation and PTSD was found mediated by depression,[11] suggesting that screening for depression in patients with PTSD may help identify those at risk for suicidality.

Chronic Disease, Physical Function, and Performance

Although the mechanism of PTSD is not known, it has been hypothesized that trauma-related alterations in autonomic reactivity, such as elevated sympathetic arousal as well as hypothalamic-pituitary-adrenal axis changes, could theoretically confer risk of cardiovascular disease. A prospective cohort study examined whether diagnosis of PTSD preceded cardiovascular disease in a male veteran population without cardiovascular disease. Veterans were assessed every 3 years to 5 years for measures of cardiovascular disease, including angina as well as fatal and nonfatal myocardial infarction. For every SD of level of PTSD symptomatology, researchers found a significant age-adjusted relative risk of 1.26 for myocardial infarction and 1.21 for all cardiovascular outcomes. The relationship was maintained when controlling for depression.[12]

PTSD also may be associated with other chronic illnesses. A study of more than 9000 individuals ages 60 years or older examined PTSD and trauma exposure through face-to-face diagnostic interviews, adjusting for sociodemographic factors and comorbid psychiatric disorders. Respondents with lifetime PTSD were more likely to have been diagnosed with hypertension, angina, heart disease, gastrointestinal ulcers, gastritis, and arthritis (OR 1.3–1.8) compared with controls.[13] Some conditions, such as gastritis and arthritis, were also seen at higher rates in those with trauma exposure but did not meet full criteria for PTSD.[13] Across studies looking at age-related medical conditions in patients with PTSD compared with those without PTSD, the most positive associations were with cardiovascular disease, type 2 diabetes mellitus, and gastrointestinal disease.[14]

PTSD is also associated with adverse effects of physical function and performance. An older veteran population with obesity was directly assessed for physical performance and the veterans provided self-reports of their function. PTSD was positively associated with worsening physical performance by self-report as well as some measures of physical function, even after controlling for demographic and other psychiatric disorders.[15]

Premature Senescence

The relationship between PTSD with age-related chronic illnesses has led to the hypothesis that PTSD may be more broadly associated with early or accelerated aging. Decreased telomere length, increased markers of oxidative stress, increased incidence of diseases associated with aging, and mortality (hazard ratio [HR] 1.29) have been seen in patients with PTSD compared with those without PTSD.[15] In another study, telomere length was negatively correlated with sexual assault and childhood trauma compared with combat trauma.[16] It is unclear if PTSD itself mediates the association with premature aging, for example, via stress-related cortisol changes as 1 possible mechanism, or if other health-related behaviors that are more common in people with PTSD, such as tobacco use, confer the relationship.

Dementia

There are increasing data to support a role for PTSD in the development of dementia. In a stratified, retrospective cohort study of more than 180,000 veterans (mean age 68.8 years) without dementia, those with a diagnosis of PTSD had an approximately 2-fold risk of developing dementia over a 7-year period compared with controls (HR 2.41; CI, 2.24–2.39). This relationship was maintained when those with a history of head injury, depression, or substance use disorder were excluded.[17] Another large retrospective cohort study of more than 10,000 veterans (65 years and older) examined rates of dementia, controlling for injury by accounting for Purple Heart status. Veterans with PTSD developed dementia with an OR of 2.2 (CI, 1.8–2.6) compared with veterans without PTSD, and this was not mediated by injury.[18] Both studies involved primarily male veterans.

The unique trauma of being a prisoner of war (POW) may also contribute to risk of dementia. Using retrospective cohort design, more than 180,000 veterans ages 55 and older were followed for a 9-year period and assessed for interactions between POW status, PTSD, and dementia. After adjustments for medical and psychiatric comorbidities as well as competing risks of dementia and death, risk of dementia was increased in the PTSD-only group (HR 1.52; CI, 1.41–1.94) and in the POW-only group (HR 1.61; CI, 1.30–1.98). Those veterans who were both POWs and had PTSD were at greatest risk of dementia, with HR 2.24 (CI, 1.72–2.92). This suggests that POW status contributes to risk of dementia with PTSD in an additive, independent manner.[19]

To further understand the impact of PTSD on cognition, 535 neurologically intact veterans with PTSD were assessed with cognitive function tests. Compared with controls, veterans with PTSD demonstrated significantly worse processing speed, verbal learning, verbal recognition, and category fluency; however, the statistical association could be attributed to modifiable factors including depression, vascular risk, and health behaviors, such as substance use and exercise.[20]

The relationship between PTSD and cognition may be reciprocal. Case studies have suggested possible worsening of PTSD symptomatology with onset of cognitive deficits on examinations and correlated with features consistent with a degenerative process on neuroimaging.[21]

Impact of remote trauma on the elderly

PTSD arising from trauma in childhood through early adulthood can theoretically have a variety of trajectories as a function of advancing age. PTSD symptoms could continue without alteration, improve, worsen, or reemerge with age. From a life course perspective, it has been hypothesized that trauma-based symptoms are expressed as a function of interactions between biological factors and accumulated individual exposures, within the context of specific communities.[22] In this model, the expression of trauma pathology is determined by the variation of the factors and their interactions. It is theorized that trauma-based symptoms may emerge or worsen in the context of aging-related challenges. Some of these stressors could include changes in roles, retirement, loss of family members and friends, loss of autonomy, and physical and cognitive decline.[23]

PTSD can persist throughout the life span. Study of veterans with PTSD arising from combat experience greater than 30 years prior reveals that many continue to experience PTSD symptoms.[24,25] In a prospective study of veterans ages 55 and older, PTSD symptom severity was assessed in 2011 and in 2013. Almost 10% of older veterans had exacerbated PTSD symptoms (compared between 2013 and 2011) arising from traumas that occurred approximately 3 decades prior. Using regression models, exacerbation could be predicted by greater cognitive impairment, specifically executive dysfunction, in 2011. The number of traumatic events since first wave and level of social support did not predict an exacerbation.[26]

Noncombat traumas can also lead to chronic PTSD. In a study of community dwellers with a mean age of 60 years, participants self-reported traumatic life events and completed PTSD and personality inventories. Cumulative trauma exposure positively correlated with PTSD symptom severity. This relationship was strongest with PTSD resulting from childhood violence and adult physical assault. PTSD was also correlated with the neurotic traits.[27] Elderly Germans examined 60 years after the end of World War II demonstrated increased rates of PTSD and subthreshold PTSD with increasing age. Posttraumatic symptoms were associated with increased rates of depressive and somatoform disorders. This suggests the effects of trauma can persist over decades and contribute to comorbid psychiatric disorders.[28] It is not known which factors maintain trauma-based symptoms over time. Attachment theorists have hypothesized that severity of trauma predicts insecure attachment in middle age and worsened PTSD symptoms in later adulthood.[29]

Possible Mechanisms Underlying the Association of Dementia and Posttraumatic Stress Disorder

The mechanism of worsening cognition in PTSD is largely unknown. It is possible that factors that determine who develops PTSD after a trauma are shared with those associated with the development of dementia. Stress hormones, including glucocorticoids, can affect cognitive performance via their effects on the hippocampus. Mouse models of Alzheimer disease exposed to trauma were found more vulnerable to PTSD, and exposure to trauma further exacerbated Alzheimer disease pathogenesis. The effects were dependent on corticotropin-releasing factor receptor 1 signaling.[30]

The €4 allele of the apolipoprotein (apoE) gene is associated with dementia and recovery from brain damage from head trauma. Using a gene-environment interaction approach, Vietnam veterans were assessed for PTSD as a function of combat exposure and apoE genotype. The gene interaction between combat and the apoE €4 allele was found to be significant for PTSD symptoms and diagnosis, suggesting that the €4 allele reduces resiliency to both physical and psychological insults.[31]

It is possible that PTSD is associated with other factors that correlate with dementia and it is not a specific independent risk factor. A cross-sectional study of older veterans with and without PTSD showed that poorer executive function and verbal learning were associated with comorbid metabolic syndrome and not mediated by PTSD.[32]

Psychotropic medications may be associated with increased risk of dementia in patients with PTSD. A retrospective cohort study followed more than 400,000 veterans older than 56 years old for 9 years with examination of psychotropic use (after PTSD diagnosis) for at least 6 months during a 3-year baseline period. As in prior studies, PTSD diagnosis was significantly associated with risk of dementia, with an HR of 1.35. Those diagnosed with PTSD and prescribed selective serotonin reuptake inhibitors (SSRIs), serotonin-norepinephrine reuptake inhibitor (SNRIs), or atypical antipsychotics were at highest risk of dementia. The investigators were not able to control for severity of illness, psychiatric comorbidity (because depression is also associated with increased risk of dementia), or other effects relating to the medications.[33]

TREATMENT OF POSTTRAUMATIC STRESS DISORDER IN THE ELDERLY

PTSD is typically treated with medication, psychotherapy, or both. Antidepressants, such as SSRIs and SNRIs, are most commonly used to treat trauma-based symptoms. Prazosin, an α_1-antagonist that crosses the blood-brain barrier, is often prescribed for hypertension and benign prostatic hypertrophy and has efficacy in targeting nightmares. In general, starting with lower doses, slower titration, and possible dose adjustment for concurrent hepatic or renal failure should be considered when treating PTSD in the elderly.

Certain medications may confer increased risk in the elderly and should be avoided or used with caution. Older antidepressants, such as tricyclics, may cause intolerable side effects due to anticholinergic properties and have more cardiac concerns. Patients with bradycardia may not tolerate prazosin at doses needed to target nightmares. Antipsychotics and benzodiazepines are believed to have limited utility in PTSD and may confer risk that is exacerbated with age. Antipsychotics carry a black box warning for all-cause mortality in the elderly with dementia. Given the risk of dementia with PTSD, the risks of antipsychotics need to be weighed against any potential benefits. Benzodiazepines are not recommended for treatment of PTSD regardless of age because they can worsen dissociation, reduce ability to engage in psychotherapy, and worsen mood and substance use.[34] In the elderly, benzodiazepines confer significant risks of falls, delirium, dependence, increased confusion, and respiratory depression and may prolong PTSD symptoms.

Derivatives of cognitive-behavioral therapy, such as prolonged exposure, and cognitive processing therapy, have significant impact on treating PTSD. There are fewer data distinguishing treatment of PTSD in the elderly compared with a younger cohort. Psychotherapy in the elderly may be less feasible because of cognitive concerns or due to limitations relating to resources or comorbidities that limit mobility and accessibility of care. Despite this, psychotherapy should be offered when indicated.

Managing Comorbid Posttraumatic Stress Disorder and Dementia

Caring for patients with both PTSD and dementia may provide added challenges. Caregivers of veterans with dementia and PTSD, compared with dementia alone, reported more challenging behavioral symptoms and more difficulties understanding veterans' memory concerns and used more community resources.[35] Elderly patients with PTSD and dementia were found at more than twice the odds of receiving second-generation antipsychotics than those with PTSD alone.[36] It is not clear, however, whether this reflects prescribing targeting symptoms PTSD or dementia or an interaction of the 2 conditions, because there was no dementia-only control group. It is possible that patients with comorbid PTSD and dementia exhibit more hypervigilance and paranoia expressed as agitation compared with a non-PTSD control group with dementia.

The Medically Ill Patient with Posttraumatic Stress Disorder

PTSD can be associated with risk of both psychiatric and medical comorbidities; however, the relationship may also be reciprocal. Case studies suggest that medical illness can exacerbate PTSD symptoms in combat veterans.[37] Conditions that alter oxygenation, such as chronic obstructive pulmonary disease, may be associated with psychological distress. Similarly, β-agonists or atrial fibrillation can cause autonomic changes that are appraised as anxiety.

Patients with PTSD who are admitted to the hospital may find the setting particularly challenging. The hospital environment is designed to provide necessary care depending on the medical situation. This can include multiple interruptions throughout the day and night for vital signs or other procedures. Patients with significant hypervigilance and hyperstartle response can be triggered with the frequent interruptions by multiple care providers. Certain necessities, including bed baths, urinary catheter changes, and incontinence care, are intimate and uncomfortable regardless of PTSD. Patients with a history of sexual trauma may feel particularly vulnerable and demonstrate exacerbations of PTSD symptoms when receiving such care.

The ICU may be uniquely challenging for patients with PTSD. Critically ill patients may not be able to respond due to sedation or weakness and are vulnerable and dependent on medical care. Aging is a significant risk factor for delirium that can be associated with the precipitation of PTSD; however, there are few data examining any possible interactions between delirious behaviors and premorbid PTSD. Anecdotally, patients with combat PTSD seen for delirium on a consult service often have features of flashbacks incorporated into their delirium manifesting as paranoia and agitation.

SUMMARY

Although PTSD is not conventionally considered a disorder of aging, it is a condition that can persist across the life span. Age-related stresses and life transitions may exacerbate PTSD symptoms, although for some patients, symptoms remit. It is unclear whether age confers a vulnerability or protective factor for trauma sustained in the elderly. Early life trauma likely has an impact on how trauma is experienced in older age.

Chronic PTSD is associated with age-related conditions, including cardiovascular disease, gastrointestinal disease, arthritis, and dementia. There are data to suggest that chronic PTSD may be associated with premature aging. Treating PTSD in the elderly may require attention to comorbidities and side effects of medications with avoidance of benzodiazepines and antipsychotics. Although patients may not specifically report trauma-based symptoms, it is important to screen for mood and trauma symptoms in the elderly.

The study of PTSD is problematic and challenging. The methodology is frequently limited by a retrospective approach or using specific populations, such as male veterans and POWs. Studies are frequently underpowered to examine relationships between developmental timing of traumatic event and the nature of the stressor. Premorbid functioning may not be able to be determined. Studies that exclude comorbid psychiatric illnesses, such as depression, may reduce the variability in data but may limit the generalizability of the results. Further research is necessary to understand the impact of timing, specific type of trauma, and cumulative effects of trauma on individuals as they age and in the elderly.

REFERENCES

1. American Psychiatric Association. Diagnostic and statistical manual of mental disorders. 5th edition. Washington, DC: 2013.
2. Palgi Y, Glkopf M, Berger R. The inoculating role of previous exposure to potentially traumatic life events on coping with prolonged exposure to rocket attacks: a lifespan perspective. Psychiatry Res 2015;227(2–3):296–301.
3. Sachs-Ericcson N, Joiner TE, Cougle JR, et al. Combat exposure in early adulthood interacts with recent stressors to predict PTSD in aging male veterans. Gerontologist 2016;56(1):82–91.
4. Chung MC, Werrett J, Easthope Y, et al. Coping with post-traumatic stress: young, middle-aged and elderly comparisons. Int J Geriatr Psychiatry 2004;19: 333–43.
5. Franco M. Posttraumatic stress disorder in older women. J Women Aging 2007; 19(1/2):103–17.
6. Breslau N, Kessler RC, Chilcoat HD, et al. Trauma and posttraumatic stress disorder in the community. Arch Gen Psychiatry 1998;55:626–32.
7. Lindbloom EJ, Brandt J, Hough LD, et al. Elder mistreatment in the nursing home: a systematic review. J Am Med Dir Assoc 2007;8(9):610–6.
8. Drews T, Franck M, Radtke FM, et al. Postoperative delirium is an independent risk factor for posttraumatic stress disorder in the elderly patient. Eur J Anaesthesiol 2015;32:147–51.
9. Barak Y, Aizenberg D, Szor H, et al. Increased risk of attempted suicide among aging holocaust survivors. Am J Geriatr Psychiatry 2005;13(8):701–4.
10. Fanning JR, Pietrzak RH. Suicidality among older male veterans in the United States: results from the National Health and Resilience in Veterans study. J Psychiatr Res 2013;47:1766–75.
11. Glaesmer H, Braehler E. The differential roles of trauma, posttraumatic stress disorder and comorbid depressive disorders on suicidal ideation in the elderly population. J Clin Psychiatry 2012;73(8):1141–6.
12. Kubzansky LD, Koenen KC, Spiro A, et al. Prospective study of posttraumatic stress disorder symptoms and coronary heart disease in the normative aging study. Arch Gen Psychiatry 2007;64:109–16.
13. Pietrzak RH, Goldstein RB, Southwick SM, et al. Physical health conditions associated with posttraumatic stress disorder in US older adults: results from Wave 2 of the National epidemiologic survey on alcohol and related conditions. J Am Geriatr Soc 2012;60(2):296–303.
14. Lohr JB, Palmer BW, Eidt CA, et al. Is post-traumatic stress disorder associated with premature senescence? A review of the literature. Am J Geriatr Psychiatry 2015;23(7):709–25.
15. Hall KS, Beckham JC, Bosworth HB, et al. PTSD is negatively associated with physical performance and physical function in older overweight military veterans. J Rehabil Res Dev 2014;51(2):285–96.
16. Li X, Wang J, Zhou J, et al. The association between post-traumatic stress disorder and shorter telomere length: a systematic review and meta-analysis. J Affect Disord 2017;218:322–6.

17. Yaffe K, Vittinghoff E, Lindquist K, et al. Posttraumatic stress disorder and risk of dementia among US veterans. Arch Gen Psychiatry 2014;67(6):608–13.
18. Quereshi SU, Kimbrell T, Pyne JM, et al. Greater Prevalence and Incidence of dementia in older veterans with Posttraumatic stress disorder. J Am Geriatr Soc 2010;58:1627–33.
19. Meziab O, Kirby KA, Williams B, et al. Prisoner of war status, posttraumatic stress disorder, and dementia in older veterans. Alzheimers Dement 2014; 14:S236–41.
20. Cohen BE, Neylan TC, Yaffe K, et al. Posttraumatic stress disorder and cognitive function: findings from the Mind Your Heart study. J Clin Psychiatry 2013;74(11): 1063–70.
21. Mittal D, Torres R, Abashidze A. Worsening of Post-traumatic stress disorder with cognitive decline: case series. J Geriatr Psychiatry Neurol 2001;14:17–20.
22. Fink DS, Galea S. Life course epidemiology of trauma and related psychopathology in civilian populations. Curr Psychiatry Rep 2015;17(5):31.
23. Davison EH, Kaiser AP, Spiro A, et al. From late-onset stress symptomatology to later-adulthood trauma reengagement in aging combat veterans: taking a broader view. Gerontologist 2016;56(1):14–21.
24. Hamilton JD, Workman RH. Persistence of combat-related posttraumatic stress symptoms for 75 years. J Trauma Stress 1998;11(4):763–8.
25. Goldberg J, Magruder KM, Forsberg CW, et al. Prevalence of Post-traumatic stress disorder in aging Vietnam-era veterans: veterans administration cooperative study 569: course and consequences of Post-traumatic stress disorder in Vietnam-era veteran twins. Am J Geriatr Psychiatry 2016;24(3): 181–91.
26. Mota N, Tsai J, Kirwin PD, et al. Late-life exacerbation of PTSD symptoms in US veterans: results from the National Health and Resilience in veterans study. J Clin Psychiatry 2016;77(3):348–54.
27. Ogle CM, Rubin DC, Siegler IC. Cumulative exposure to traumatic events in older adults. Aging Ment Health 2014;18(3):316–25.
28. Glaesmer H, Kaiser M, Braehler E, et al. Posttraumatic stress disorder and its co-morbidity with depression and somatization in the elderly – A German community-based study. Aging Ment Health 2012;16(4):403–12.
29. Franz CE, Lyons MJ, Spoon KM, et al. Post-traumatic stress symptoms and adult attachment: a 24 year long longitudinal study. Am J Geriatr Psychiatry 2014; 22(12):1603–12.
30. Justice NJ, Huang L, Tian JB, et al. Posttraumatic stress disorder-like induction elevated β-amyloid levels, which directly activates corticotropin-releasing factor neurons to exacerbate the stress the responses. J Neurosci 2015;35(6): 2612–23.
31. Lyons MJ, Genderson M, Grant MD, et al. Gene-environment interaction of ApoE genotype and combat exposure on PTSD. Am J Med Genet B Neuropsychiatr Genet 2013;162B(7):762–9.
32. Green E, Fairchild JK, Kinoshita LM, et al. Effects of posttraumatic stress disorder and metabolic syndrome on cognitive aging in veterans. Gerontologist 2016; 56(1):72–81.
33. Mawanda F, Wallace RB, McCoy K, et al. PTSD, psychotropic medication use and risk of dementia among US veterans: a retrospective cohort study. J Am Geriatr Soc 2017;65(5):1043–50.
34. Guina J, Rossetter SR, DeRhodes BJ, et al. Benzodiazepines for PTSD: a systematic review and meta-analysis. J Psychiatr Pract 2015;21(4):281–303.

35. Pinciotti CM, Bass DM, McCarthy CA, et al. Negative consequences of family caregiving for veterans with PTSD and dementia. J Nerv Ment Dis 2017;205(2): 106–11.
36. Semla TP, Lee A, Gurrera R, et al. Off-label prescribing of second-generation antipsychotics to elderly veterans with posttraumatic stress disorder and dementia. J Am Geriatr Soc 2017;65(8):1789–95.
37. Hamner MB. Exacerbation of Posttraumatic stress disorder symptoms with medical illness. Gen Hosp Psychiatry 1994;16:135–7.

Printed and bound by CPI Group (UK) Ltd, Croydon, CR0 4YY

07/10/2024

01040503-0014